TURMERIC
A COOKBOOK

First published in Great Britain in 2017
by Aster, an imprint of
Octopus Publishing Group Ltd
Carmelite House
50 Victoria Embankment
London EC4Y 0DZ
www.octopusbooks.co.uk

An Hachette UK Company
www.hachette.co.uk

The authorized representative in the EEA
is Hachette Ireland, 8 Castlecourt Centre,
Dublin 15, D15 XTP3, Ireland
(email: info@hbgi.ie)

This edition published in 2026

Copyright © Octopus Publishing
Group Ltd 2017, 2026

Distributed in the US by Hachette Book
Group
1290 Avenue of the Americas
4th and 5th Floors, New York, NY 10104

Distributed in Canada by Canadian
Manda Group, 664 Annette St.,
Toronto, Ontario, Canada M6S 2C8

All rights reserved. No part of this work
may be reproduced or utilized in any
form or by any means, electronic or
mechanical, including photocopying,
recording or by any information storage
and retrieval system, without the prior
written permission of the publisher.

ISBN: 978-0-6006-4008-0
eISBN: 978-0-6006-4009-7

A CIP catalogue record for this book
is available from the British Library.

Printed and bound in China.

10 9 8 7 6 5 4 3 2 1

Publisher: Lucy Pessell
Senior Editor: Tim Leng
Designers: Isobel Platt & Kath Anderson
Assistant Editor: Samina Rahman
Production Controller: Allison Gonsalves

Photographer: Issy Croker
Props Stylist: Emily Ezekiel
Page 7 picture credit: Wellcome Library,
London

This FSC® label means that materials
used for the product have been
responsibly sourced.

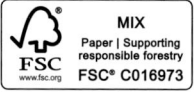

TURMERIC
A COOKBOOK

Breakfast – lunch – dinner
and everything in between

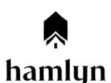

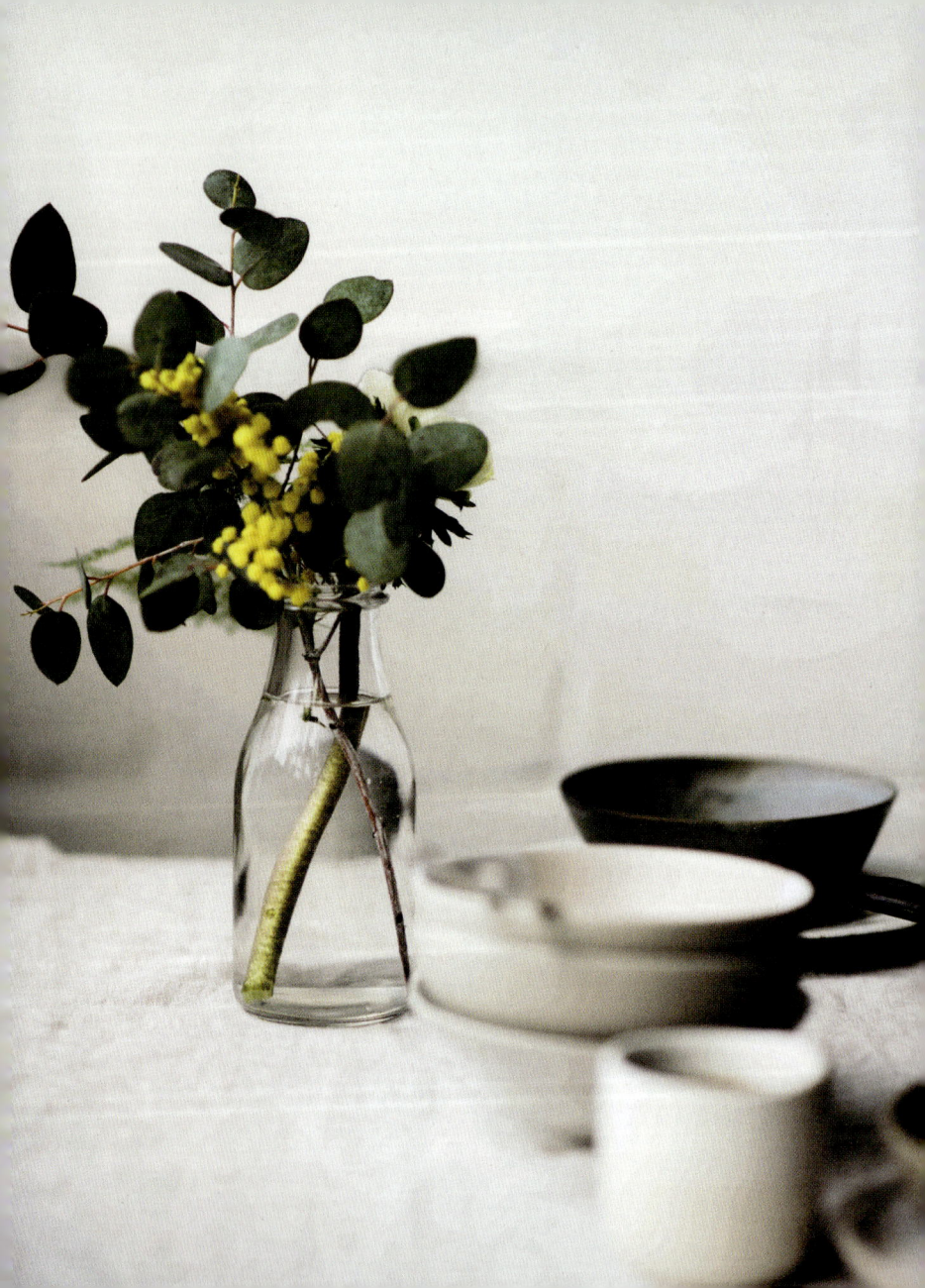

CONTENTS

6 Introduction

10 **Breakfasts**

18 **Soups, sides & snacks**

44 **Main dishes**

66 **Sweets & drinks**

78 Index

INTRODUCTION

Turmeric, the spice best known as an ingredient in curries, is one of nature's most powerful ancient healers and has been used medicinally for over 4,500 years. It comes from the root of *Curcuma longa*, a green plant in the ginger family, and is grown throughout the tropics, especially in India and Indonesia. On the island of Bali, turmeric is at the heart of their traditional medicine, and 'Jamu' tonics are widely available to cure your ailments and boost your well-being.

Turmeric appears in some of the earliest known records of plant medicines. It is mentioned in Egyptian texts and is thought to have been cultivated in the Hanging Gardens of Babylon, one of the Seven Wonders of the Ancient World. In India, turmeric plays an important part in Ayurvedic medicine, originating around 2,500 years ago. Inhaling the fumes from burning turmeric was said to alleviate congestion; turmeric paste or juice was used to heal wounds and bruises; and the spice was also used for digestive issues.

Modern medicine is now beginning to confirm many of the reported health benefits of turmeric, especially its anti-cancer properties. Much of the research is focused on one of the main components of turmeric, a substance called curcumin. However, attention is now also being directed at studying the effects of the whole root and the pages that follow will explore all the potential health benefits of this wonder root.

COOKING WITH TURMERIC

So, we are all starting to hear more about turmeric and how it might be a good idea to include plenty of it in our diets. But beyond curry, how do we do that?

As it happens, alongside the increased attention of the medical community, chefs and healthy foodies have been trying out turmeric in an amazing array of dishes. Traditional 'golden milks' and tonics are growing in popularity; turmeric teas and turmeric honey are now available; and supermarkets are beginning to sell the fresh root alongside ginger, as well as in its ground or powdered form.

Turmeric has a very individual taste that is difficult to describe, except to say it is quite pungent and bitter. However, when combined with other flavours, its culinary use widens considerably; for example, it goes well with honey so can be used in desserts, on top of porridge or in granola. You can also use it in baking, roasting vegetables, in salad dressings or even in ice cream.

And as turmeric has anti-ageing properties, it can also be used as a natural beauty ingredient, so we've included some different face masks to try and a homemade turmeric soap.

> *'Each spice has a special day to it. For turmeric it is Sunday, when light drips fat and butter-coloured into the bins to be soaked up glowing, when you pray to the nine planets for love and luck.'*
>
> – Chitra Banerjee Divakaruni, *The Mistress of Spices*

ANCIENT HEALER, MODERN MEDICINE

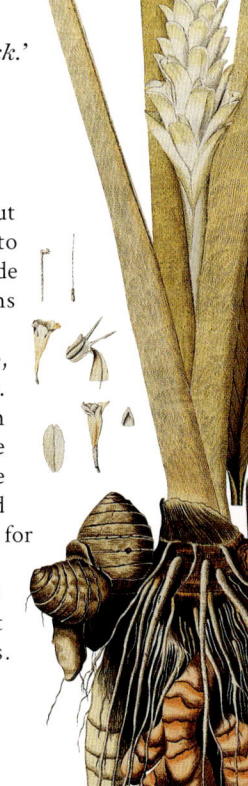

While the Assyrians and the ancient Greeks knew about and used turmeric, it is Asian herbalists – likely due to turmeric needing tropical conditions to thrive – who made the most medicinal use of this spice until the Europeans began to catch up in the late 20th century.

In Ayurveda, the Indian system of herbal medicine, turmeric is thought to 'strengthen and warm' the body. It is used specifically to improve the digestive system and microbiome, to regulate menstruation, relieve the inflammation associated with arthritis, and balance the metabolism. It is also used as an anti-inflammatory and antibacterial agent for coughs and colds, and on the skin for burns, cuts and bruises.

The ancient Hawaiians are also thought to have used turmeric for ear and sinus infections, most probably due to the spice's astringent properties.

And across Indonesia, the recipes for turmeric tonics are still closely guarded family secrets. They are used in the traditional herbal healing system known as Jamu both for general preventative well-being and for the treatment of specific conditions, such as joint pain.

In Europe, serious research on the health properties of turmeric began in Germany in the 1920s, and in the 1960s its benefits to the digestive system started to be discussed. By the 1990s, turmeric was being more regularly recommended by Western herbalists, and today doctors and general practitioners often recommend turmeric as part of a healthy diet, especially for cancer patients.

Research into the heart benefits of turmeric has focused on curcumin, its main active ingredient. This has been shown to have anti-inflammatory effects, and it is also an antioxidant. Inflammation has been linked to heart disease, diabetes, Alzheimer's, stroke and cancer. Antioxidants protect the body from the damage caused by free radicals, which we are exposed to through normal bodily processes, such as digestion and burning sugars for energy, and through our environment. The anti-inflammatory and antioxidant effects of turmeric are also believed to benefit overall health and well-being when included in a healthy diet.

Recently, studies have shown the potential anti-cancer benefits of turmeric, specifically when consumed through cooking. It is thought that it may be helpful both as part of a preventative lifestyle and for cancer patients undergoing treatment.

DOSAGE

It is currently thought that about a teaspoon of fresh or ground turmeric a day is helpful for promoting gut health and general wellness.

TURMERIC AND BLACK PEPPER

Black pepper contains the compound piperine which helps increase absorption of curcumin. It isn't always necessary to consume turmeric with black pepper, but it has been shown to boost the body's ability to absorb the beneficial properties.

PREPARATION AND USES

The ground turmeric that we easily recognize from its bright orange colour comes from the 'fingers' that grow from the root. The root is cleaned and boiled then dried at a low temperature before being processed into a powder. Turmeric can also be used in a similar way to fresh root ginger, grated directly into recipes or infused in oils (see page 43) or in hot water for tea. Turmeric root now more readily available in supermarkets and delis has a slightly sweeter taste than the powder.

Turmeric can be eaten both raw and cooked. For example, you can grate it into dressings, ice cream or tonics (see pages 36, 49 and 69), or add a little to soups and stews (see pages 19, 23 and 26).

WHEN EVERYTHING TURNS YELLOW

The only problem with turmeric is that it can easily discolour your pots and pans, your worktops and even your hands. Lemon juice or white vinegar can remove the colouring, or for more stubborn stains you can use a bleach-based cleaner. If you spill a bit of sauce containing turmeric, you can try sprinkling the stain with talcum powder or bicarbonate of soda (baking soda) and then blotting gently with kitchen paper (paper towel). The key thing is to try not to rub it in! For clothes, sometimes bleach is the only answer, but apparently soaking the item and putting it in sunlight may help to fade the stain. And for your skin, try mixing sugar and water and gently scrubbing your hands; this works as a natural exfoliator at the same time as removing that telltale yellow hue.

BREAKFASTS

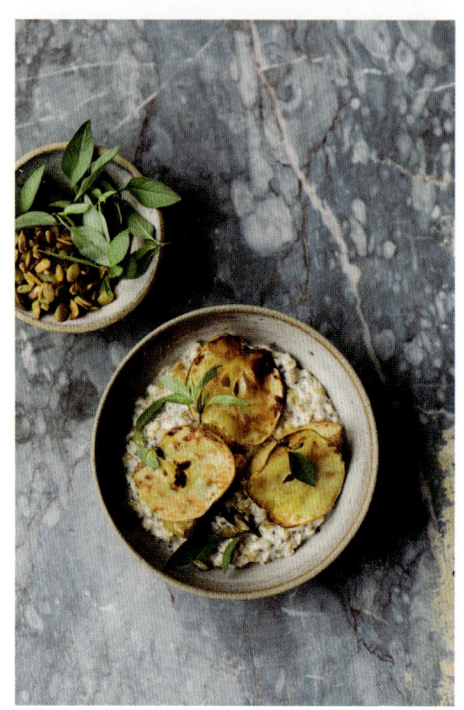

11	**Bircher Muesli**
12	**Coconut & Cashew Granola**
13	**Frittata**
14	**Devilled Scrambled Eggs**
16	**Smoked Mackerel Turmeric Congee**

SERVES 2

BIRCHER MUESLI
with turmeric honey

Soaking oats overnight makes breakfast quick and easy in the morning. You can then simply heat them up with a little extra milk or water and serve with a spoonful of turmeric honey, or turn into a Bircher muesli with some chopped fruit and nuts.

---

100 g (3½ oz) porridge (rolled) oats
1 tablespoon flaxseeds
1 tablespoon chia seeds
¼ teaspoon ground cinnamon
100 ml (3½ fl oz) unsweetened almond milk
200 ml (7 fl oz) water
few drops of vanilla extract
2 apples
juice of ½ lime
2 tablespoons natural (plain) yogurt
1 tablespoon hazelnuts, roughly chopped
1 teaspoon coconut oil (optional)

FOR THE TURMERIC HONEY
(MAKES 200 G/7 OZ)
50 g (2 oz) coconut oil
150 g (5 oz) raw clear (liquid) honey
2 teaspoons ground turmeric
¼ teaspoon ground black pepper

TO SERVE
spiced & roasted seeds (see page 30)
Thai basil leaves

First make the turmeric honey. Heat the coconut oil so that it is in liquid form. Add to a bowl with the honey, turmeric and pepper and combine thoroughly. Transfer to a glass jar and store at room temperature until needed.

The night before, mix together the oats, seeds, cinnamon, almond milk, water and vanilla extract in a large bowl and chill in the refrigerator overnight.

In the morning, grate 1 of the apples and stir into the oats with the lime juice, yogurt, chopped hazelnuts and 2 tablespoons of the turmeric honey.

Slice the remaining apple and, if liked, sauté in a little coconut oil. Use to top the Bircher muesli. Finish with a sprinkling of roasted seeds and a few Thai basil leaves, if using.

MAKES ABOUT 500 G (1 LB)

COCONUT & CASHEW GRANOLA

Making your own granola means you can put in all your favourite ingredients. The coconut flakes and cashew nuts included here create a light granola, while the honey and cinnamon add just the right amount of sweetness.

---

250 g (8 oz) jumbo oats
125 g (4 oz) raw cashew nuts, roughly chopped
50 g (2 oz) pumpkin seeds
50 g (2 oz) sunflower seeds
25 g (1 oz) golden flaxseeds
½ teaspoon ground cinnamon
½ teaspoon ground turmeric
½ teaspoon ground ginger
2 heaped tablespoons coconut oil
60 g (2½ oz) raw clear (liquid) honey
1 teaspoon vanilla extract

Preheat the oven to 140°C (275°F), Gas Mark 1 and line a large baking tray with baking paper (parchment).

Mix all the dry ingredients together in a large bowl.

Heat the coconut oil and honey in a saucepan until dissolved, then add the vanilla extract. Pour this into the dry ingredients and stir thoroughly so that all the oats, nuts and seeds are evenly coated.

Pour the granola on to the prepared tray and spread out evenly. Bake for about 1 hour, until golden and just crunchy. Allow to cool in the switched-off oven, then gently bring up the sides of the paper to transfer the granola to an airtight jar.

SERVES 2

FRITTATA

The best way to get anyone to eat more greens is to combine them with eggs and cheese. This frittata is simple but the trick is to get the heat high enough for the eggs to puff up when they hit the pan, similar to an omelette.

---

1 tablespoon coconut oil
1 teaspoon grated fresh root ginger
1 teaspoon grated fresh turmeric
200 g (7 oz) cavolo nero (black kale), stalks removed and leaves chopped
4 large eggs
knob of butter
1 tablespoon crème fraîche (sour cream)
100 g (3½ oz) sheep's milk cheese, shaved
sea salt and ground black pepper

Preheat the oven to 220°C (425°F), Gas Mark 7.

Heat the coconut oil in a small, nonstick, ovenproof frying pan (skillet). Add the ginger and turmeric and fry over a medium heat until you can smell the aroma. Add the cavolo nero, season with salt and pepper and allow to wilt. Remove from the heat, transfer to a bowl and massage the wilted leaves with your hands.

Whisk the eggs vigorously while you melt the butter in the same pan over a high heat. Stir the crème fraîche into the eggs. Once the pan is very hot and the butter is foaming, add the egg and crème fraîche mixture. The edges should puff up straight away. Add shavings of cheese and the wilted greens before transferring the pan to the oven. Cook for about 5 minutes, until the top is puffed and golden. Serve immediately.

SERVES 2

DEVILLED SCRAMBLED EGGS
with avocado on toast

Adding a few spices to your eggs makes the perfect accompaniment to avocado on toast for a great Sunday brunch.

---

4 eggs
½ teaspoon ground turmeric
¼ teaspoon hot paprika
¼ teaspoon chilli powder
6 tablespoons milk or non-dairy alternative
2 thick slices of sourdough bread
extra virgin olive oil, for drizzling
1 ripe avocado
juice of ½ lemon
2 teaspoons butter or coconut oil
good pinch of chilli flakes
sea salt flakes

Crack the eggs into a bowl and whisk in the spices and milk.

Preheat the grill (broiler). Drizzle the sourdough slices with extra virgin olive oil, sprinkle with sea salt flakes and put under the grill.

Meanwhile, cut the avocado in half and remove the stone. Scoop out the flesh and mash with the lemon juice and a little salt.

Melt the butter or coconut oil in a nonstick frying pan (skillet) over a high heat and add the eggs and a good pinch of salt. Leave for several seconds to start cooking on the bottom, then gently fold the eggs over and into one another – do not stir. Remove from the heat when still just slightly liquid.

Spread the toasted sourdough with the mashed avocado and spoon over the scrambled eggs. Sprinkle with the chilli flakes and serve immediately.

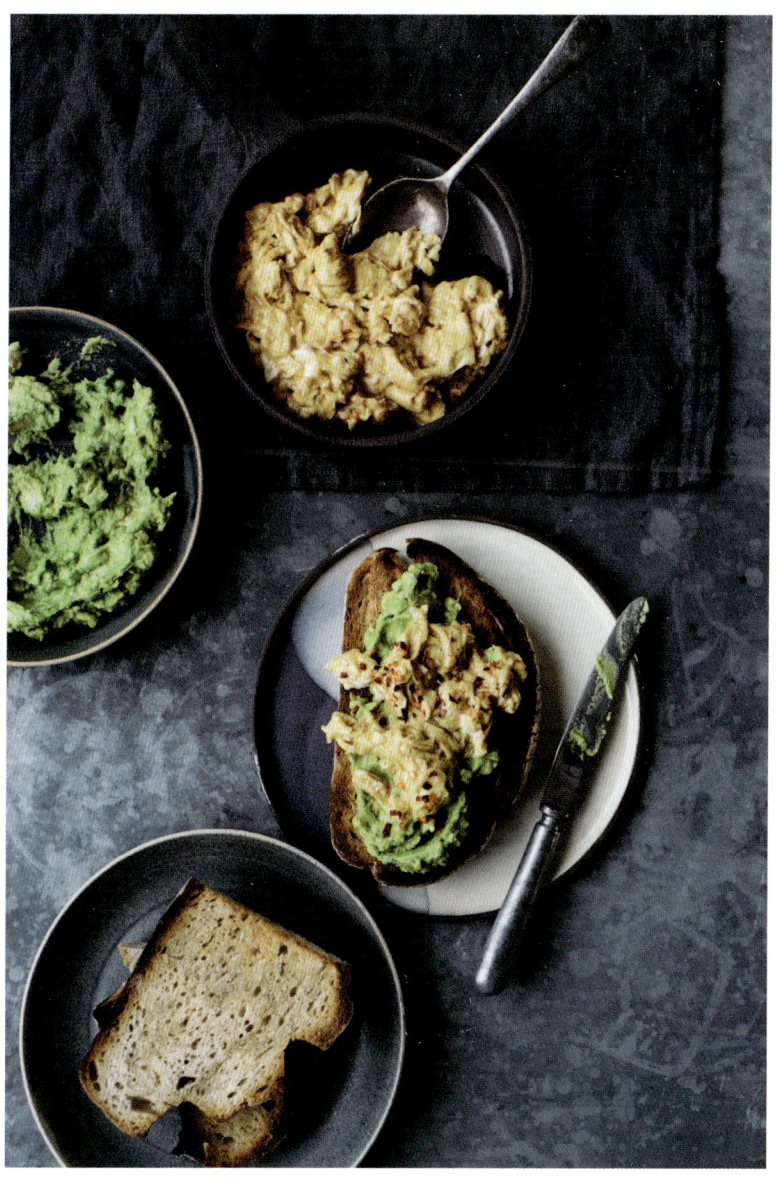

SERVES 2

SMOKED MACKEREL TURMERIC CONGEE

Congee is simply rice that has been cooked longer that usual so that it goes very soft. It's similar to risotto but comes from Asia, and is often eaten for breakfast as a kind of savoury porridge.

---

2 tablespoons sesame oil
25 g (1 oz) fresh root ginger, peeled and thinly sliced
3 garlic cloves, thinly sliced
1 teaspoon ground turmeric
200 g (7 oz) short-grain rice, washed thoroughly
4 dried shiitake mushrooms, rehydrated in warm water
450 ml (¾ pint) chicken or fish stock (broth)
450 ml (¾ pint) water
4 tablespoons light soy sauce

TO SERVE

2 eggs
1 tablespoon vinegar, for poaching
2 large smoked mackerel fillets, at room temperature
1 shallot, thinly sliced
1 radish, thinly sliced
few sprigs of lemon verbena or picked coriander (cilantro) leaves

Heat 1 tablespoon of the sesame oil in a saucepan over a medium heat and lightly fry the ginger and garlic. You don't want much colour, so fry until they're aromatic and just slightly softer. Add the turmeric and stir well.

Add the rice and the shiitake mushrooms to the pan and mix thoroughly. The mushrooms are to add a bit of background umami to the dish.

Add the stock and the water and cook for about 1 hour over a low heat, or until the rice becomes soft and porridge-like with a fair amount of liquid left in the pan. If the congee gets too dry, add more water or stock until the consistency returns. Once the rice is cooked, add the soy sauce and the other tablespoon of sesame oil.

Meanwhile, poach the eggs. Bring a saucepan of water to a rolling boil and add the vinegar. Crack the eggs into a saucer or small cup and tip gently into the water. Poach for 6 minutes, then remove with a slotted spoon and drain on kitchen paper (paper towel).

Divide the rice between two bowls and top each one with flakes of the mackerel and a poached egg. Garnish with the sliced shallot and radish, and the lemon verbena sprigs.

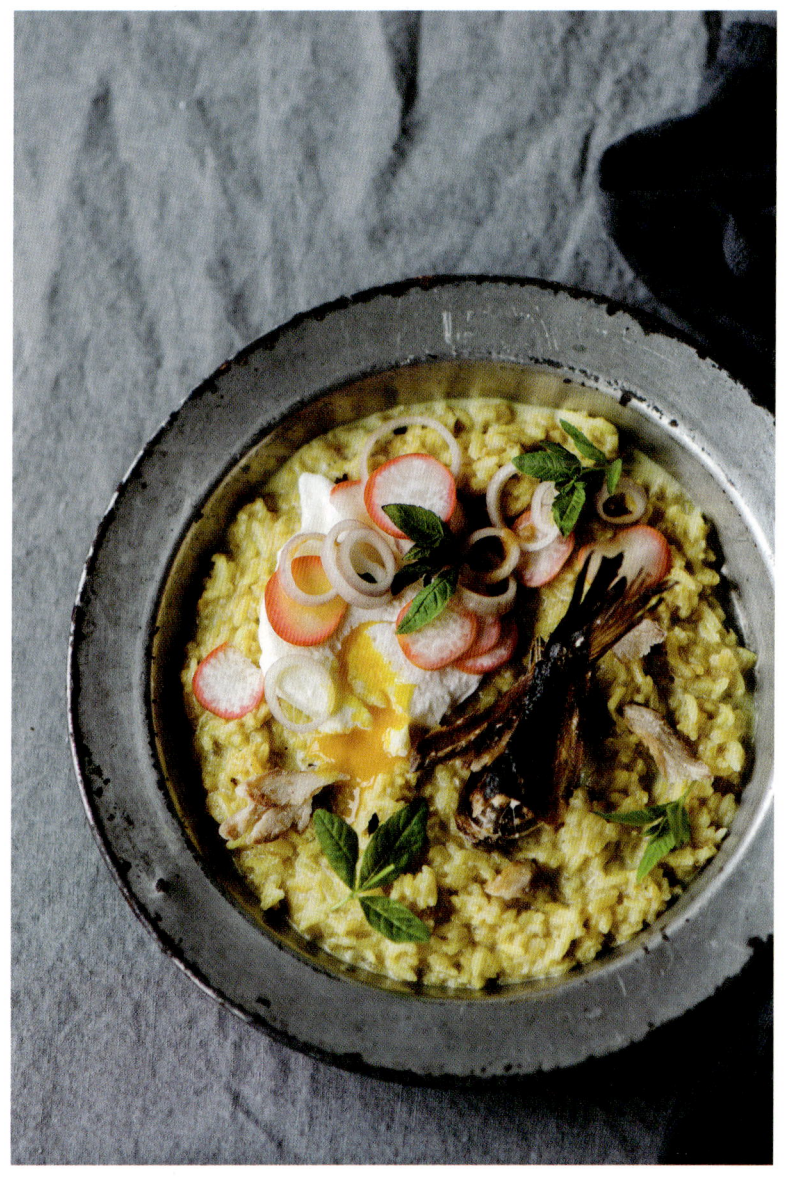

SOUPS, SIDES & SNACKS

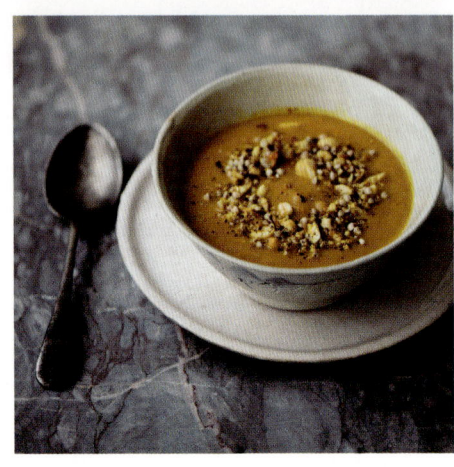

19	**Ginger & Turmeric Carrot Soup**
21	**Kitchari**
22	**Squash & Coconut Dhal**
23	**Bacon & Egg-Drop Miso**
25	**Rasam**
26	**Coconut Chicken Soup**
28	**Turmeric Bliss Balls**
30	**Spiced & Roasted Seeds**
31	**Turmeric & Black Pepper Oatcakes**
33	**Turmeric Hummus**
35	**Corn On The Cob**
36	**New Potato Salad**
39	**Roast Aubergine**
40	**Turmeric Banana Bread**
42	**Turmeric Pickles**
43	**Turmeric Mustard**
43	**Turmeric-Infused Oil**

SERVES 2

GINGER & TURMERIC CARROT SOUP

This is a quick and very tasty soup, perfect for a cold winter's day.

---

1 tablespoon groundnut (peanut) oil
½ onion, chopped
1 teaspoon grated fresh root ginger
1 teaspoon grated fresh turmeric or ground turmeric
pinch of ground black pepper, plus extra to season
250 g (8 oz) carrots, roughly chopped
400 ml (14 fl oz) hot vegetable stock (broth)
40 g (½ oz) cashew nuts, roughly chopped
½ teaspoon mild chilli powder
sea salt flakes

Heat the oil in a saucepan over a low–medium heat, add the onion and sauté for about 10 minutes, until soft. Add the ginger, turmeric and black pepper and stir through before adding the carrots.

Continue to stir the carrots for another couple of minutes, then add the stock. Bring to the boil, then reduce the heat and simmer for 10–15 minutes, or until the carrots can be easily pierced with a sharp knife.

Transfer the soup to a blender and process until smooth; taste and adjust the seasoning.

Mix the chopped cashew nuts with the mild chilli powder and dry roast in a frying pan (skillet) for a few minutes over a low heat.

Serve the soup in bowls with the spiced cashew nuts scattered over the top.

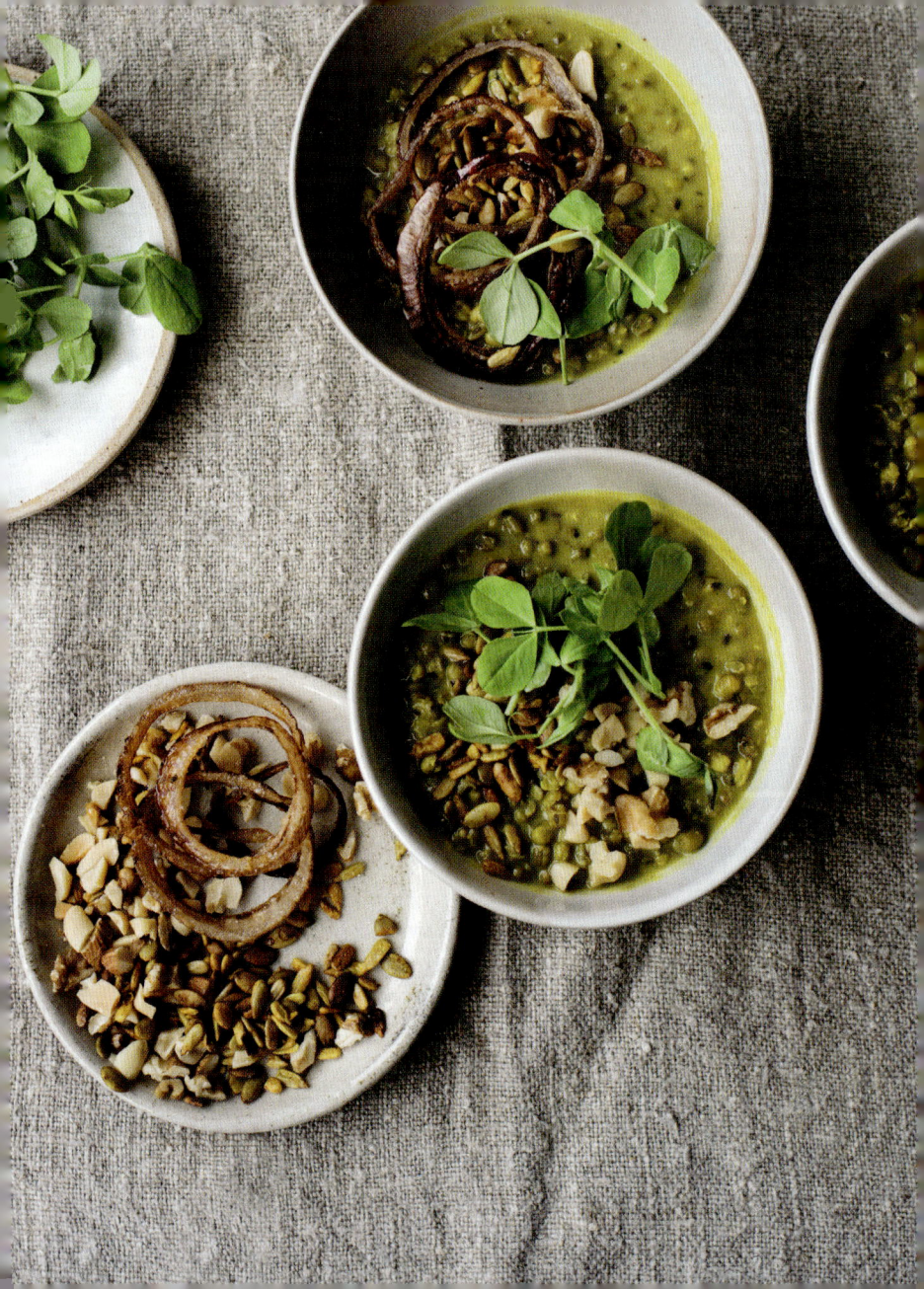

SERVES 2

KITCHARI

This recipe is based on an Ayurvedic cleansing soup; if you are doing the cleanse, you eat only kitchari for a certain number of days. We've included it as it's just a surprisingly delicious recipe.

---

100 g (3½ oz) green mung beans, rinsed and soaked overnight
1 teaspoon ground turmeric
¼ teaspoon ground black pepper
1 sheet of kombu seaweed or ¼ teaspoon asafoetida
20 g (¾ oz) butter
¼ teaspoon mustard seeds
¼ teaspoon cumin seeds
¼ teaspoon fennel seeds
¼ teaspoon nigella seeds
6 dried curry leaves
zest and juice of 1 lemon
sea salt flakes

FOR THE CRISPY ONIONS (OPTIONAL)
vegetable oil, for frying
1 onion, sliced into rings
plain (all-purpose) flour, for dusting

TO SERVE
natural (plain) yogurt
chopped nuts
spiced & roasted seeds (see page 30)
pea shoots

Rinse the mung beans a couple of times, then drain and put into a saucepan with 1 litre (1¾ pints) of water.

Add the turmeric, black pepper and seaweed or asafoetida and bring to the boil. Reduce to a low simmer and cook for about an hour, until the beans are soft.

Melt the butter in a frying pan (skillet) over a medium heat and, when bubbling, add the seeds, curry leaves and lemon zest. When the seeds begin to pop, remove from the heat and carefully add to the kitchari. Add the lemon juice and sea salt to taste.

Take the kitchari off the heat, then cover and rest for 5–10 minutes while you prepare the crispy onions, if using.

Heat the vegetable oil in a wok over a high heat. Dip the onion rings in flour and carefully lower a few at a time into the hot oil with tongs. When they are golden and crispy remove from the pan and drain on kitchen paper (paper towel).

Top the kitchari with any or all of the serving suggestions listed: crispy onions, a dollop of yogurt, some chopped nuts, roasted seeds and pea shoots.

SERVES 4

SQUASH & COCONUT DHAL

Dhal is a great standby to have during the week, and the butternut squash added here makes it a really satisfying meal in a bowl. Tamari is not an everyday companion for dhal or turmeric, but it adds a lovely flavour.

---

225 g (7½ oz) yellow split peas, rinsed and drained
600 ml (1 pint) vegetable stock
500 g (1lb) butternut squash, peeled, deseeded and diced
2 tablespoons tamari
50 g (2 oz) coconut cream
2 tablespoons olive oil
2 teaspoons mustard seeds
1 onion, thinly sliced
1 teaspoon ground turmeric

Put the split peas into a saucepan with the stock, bring to a simmer and cook gently for about 30 minutes. Add the squash, tamari and coconut cream and cook for another 15–20 minutes, until the squash is soft. If you prefer your dhal smooth, transfer to a blender and process until smooth.

Heat the olive oil in a small frying pan (skillet). Add the mustard seeds and stir until they start popping. Add the onion and soften for 10 minutes over a low–medium heat. Stir in the turmeric and cook for a few more minutes.

Ladle the dhal into bowls and top with the aromatic onions. Serve immediately.

SERVES 2

BACON & EGG-DROP MISO

This is a really quick soup, perfect for lunch or after exercising. Make it vegetarian by leaving out the bacon – it's just as good.

- 2 slices streaky (regular) bacon, chopped into small pieces
- 2 spring onions (scallions), thinly sliced
- 2 teaspoons brown miso paste
- ½ teaspoon grated fresh turmeric or ground turmeric
- 2 large handfuls of baby spinach
- 2 eggs, beaten

Heat a nonstick saucepan and fry the bacon over a medium heat, adding the spring onions after a couple of minutes.

Dissolve the miso paste in a little just-boiled water and add to the pan, along with about 500 ml (17 fl oz) just-boiled water and the turmeric. Allow the flavours to infuse for a couple of minutes before adding the spinach.

When the spinach has wilted down a little, slowly add the beaten eggs to the soup, ideally through a slotted spoon to help create ribbons.

As soon as the egg sets, remove from the heat, divide between 2 bowls and serve.

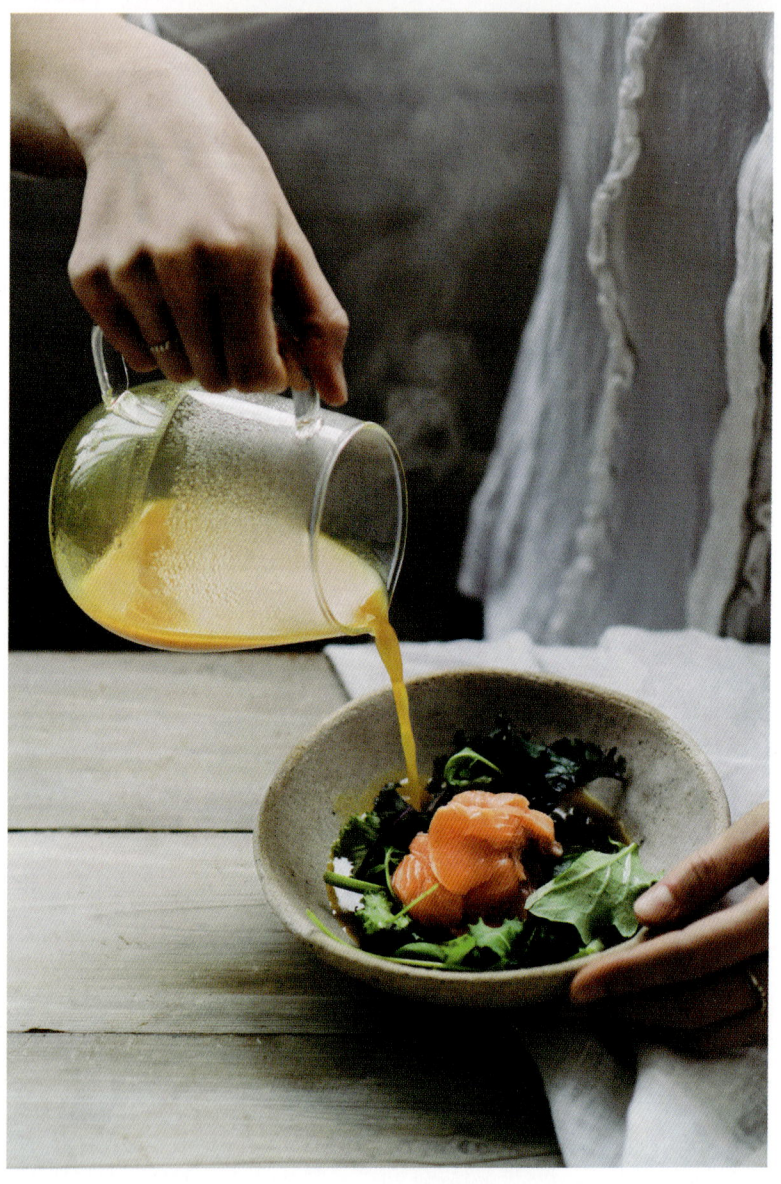

SERVES 4

RASAM
with sashimi & wilting greens

There is a bit of theatre in this dish as you pour the rasam broth over the fish and greens at the table.

---

65 g (2½ oz) tamarind paste
750 ml (1¼ pints) hot water (from a boiled kettle)
1 tomato, quartered
400 g (13 oz) good-quality skinless salmon fillet, very thinly sliced at an angle
4 tablespoons Greek yogurt
100 g (3½ oz) baby spinach
100 g (3½ oz) baby kale

FOR THE RASAM PASTE
½ teaspoon cracked black pepper
1 teaspoon ground turmeric
4 dried red chillies
1 teaspoon cumin seeds
4 garlic cloves
20 g (¾) coriander (cilantro) stems

FOR THE TEMPER
1 teaspoon coconut oil
1 teaspoon black mustard seeds
½ teaspoon cumin seeds
10–12 dried curry leaves
¼ teaspoon asafoetida

First put the tamarind paste and hot water into a large saucepan to steep for about 10 minutes.

Meanwhile, make the rasam paste by pounding all the ingredients together using a pestle and mortar until they form a coarse paste. Alternatively, you can blitz the ingredients in a blender, but the idea is to keep the paste coarse.

By this time, the tamarind should be soft. Mix the tamarind water with the rasam paste, add the tomato and place over a low–medium heat to warm through.

For the temper, heat the coconut oil in a frying pan (skillet). Add the mustard seeds and, once they start popping, add the cumin allowing it to brown slightly (30 seconds or so). Add the curry leaves and asafoetida and stir for several seconds. Add to the rasam broth, bring to the boil, then simmer for 5–6 minutes. Take off the heat and strain the rasam, pressing on the tomatoes to get all the flavour.

To serve, place a tablespoon of yogurt in each bowl. Arrange the spinach and baby kale on top, then place 3 or 4 slices of the salmon on top of the greens. Bring the rasam back to the boil, serve the bowls at the table and pour the piping hot rasam over the fish.

SERVES 2

COCONUT CHICKEN SOUP
with turmeric & kale

The sweetness of coconut goes very well with turmeric; here the use of coconut water as opposed to coconut milk creates a light, fresh and healthy soup that warms both body and soul.

---

1 tablespoon coconut oil
1 small onion, chopped
200 ml (7 fl oz) coconut water
200ml (7 fl oz) hot chicken stock (broth)
1 teaspoon grated fresh turmeric or ground turmeric
¼ teaspoon ground black pepper
100 g (3½ oz) kale, stalks removed and leaves shredded
1 baby gem lettuce, halved
1 tablespoon olive oil
100 g (3½ oz) leftover roast chicken
squeeze of lemon juice, to taste (optional)
sea salt flakes

Melt half the coconut oil in a heavy-based saucepan and sauté the onion over a medium heat until soft, about 8–10 minutes. Add the coconut water, stock, turmeric and black pepper. Keep at a low simmer.

Heat the remaining coconut oil in a frying pan (skillet) or wok and sauté the kale with a good pinch of sea salt for a few minutes, until softened.

Place a griddle pan over a high heat, brush the lettuce halves with the olive oil and griddle on both sides for 2–3 minutes.

Divide the kale, lettuce and chicken between bowls and pour over the hot coconut chicken stock. Taste and add lemon juice, if using. Serve immediately.

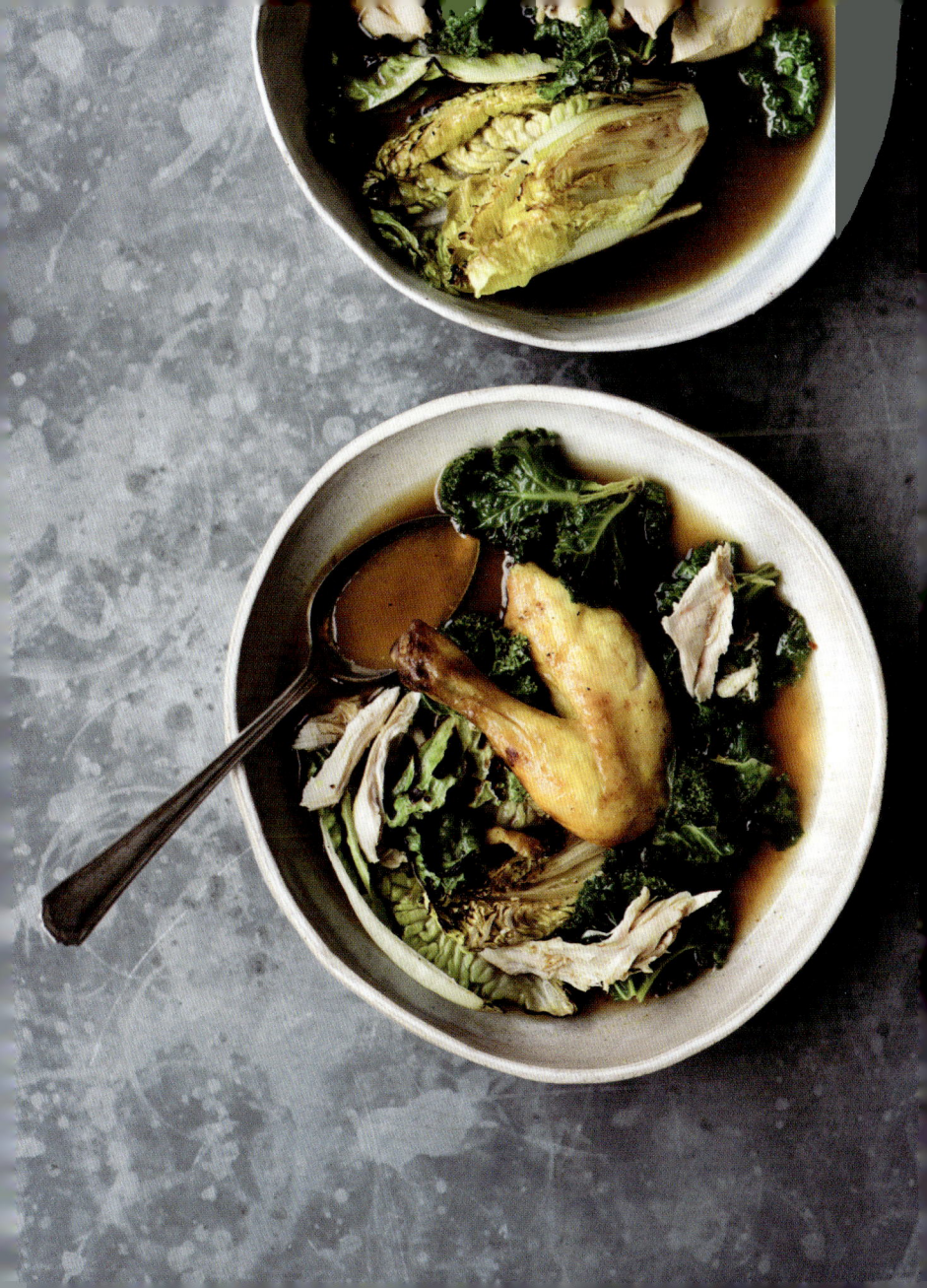

MAKES 10

TURMERIC BLISS BALLS

You can store these balls in the refrigerator for up to 5 days. They are great as a snack for when you feel like a treat or need a burst of energy, and are particularly good for days when you are exercising.

---

70 g (2½ oz) whole almonds
30 g (1 oz) flaxseeds
30 g (1 oz) desiccated (shredded) coconut, plus extra for rolling
120g dried apple, soaked in hot water for 1 minute, then drained
1 teaspoon ground turmeric
½ teaspoon ground cinnamon
1 tablespoon raw cacao powder
2 tablespoons coconut oil, melted
2 tablespoons raw clear (liquid) honey, or use the Turmeric Honey on page 11 and omit the turmeric above)

Put all the ingredients into a food processor and blend to a paste.

Roll into balls about the size of a walnut, then coat in the extra desiccated coconut.

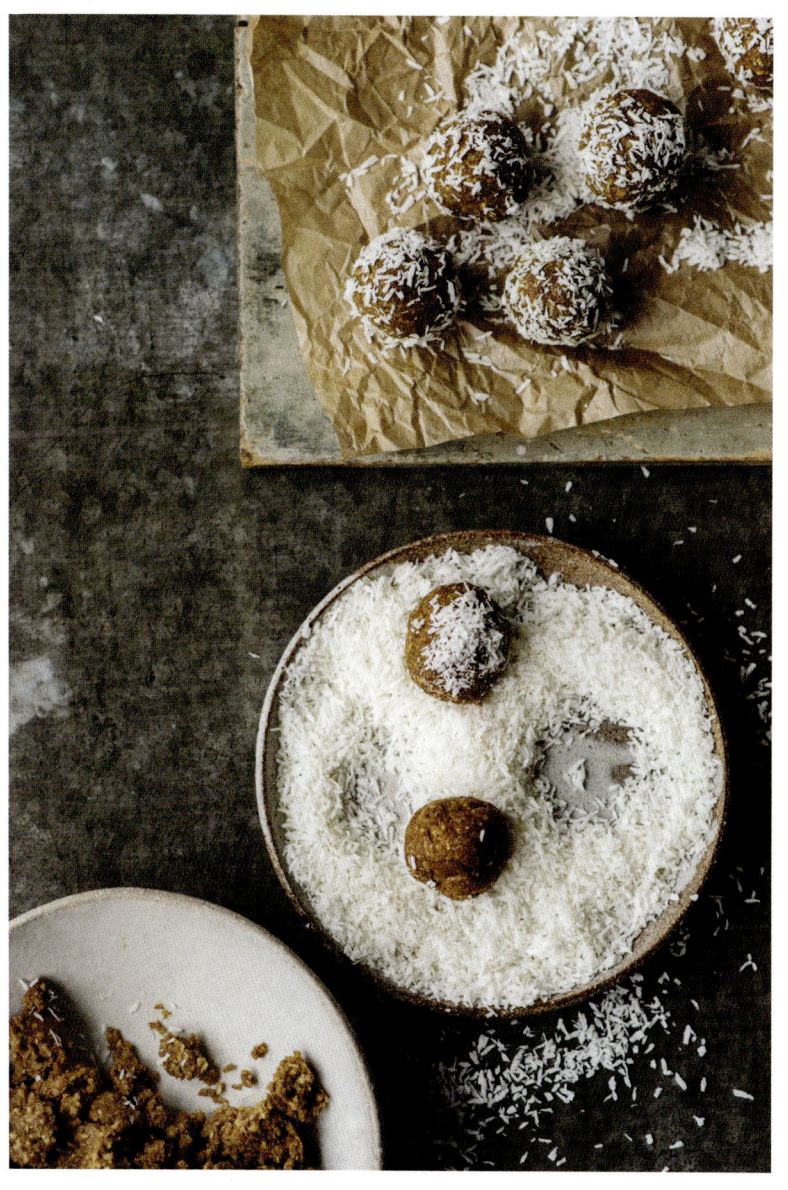

MAKES 200 G (7 OZ)

SPICED & ROASTED SEEDS

Orange juice adds a sweetness to this savoury snack. The seeds are great for taking with you when on the go, or you can use them to add a bit of crunch to soups and salads.

---

100 g (3½ oz) pumpkin seeds
100 g (3½ oz) sunflower seeds
1 tablespoon olive oil
juice of 1 lime
juice of 1 orange
½ teaspoon ground turmeric
½ teaspoon mild chilli powder
½ teaspoon sea salt flakes

Preheat the oven to 180°C (350°F), Gas Mark 4 and line a baking tray with baking paper (parchment).

Mix all the ingredients together in a bowl, then spread out over the lined tray. Roast for 30–40 minutes, shaking the seeds halfway through cooking, until golden and crunchy.

Allow to cool, then transfer to an airtight jar.

MAKES ABOUT 20 SMALL OATCAKES

TURMERIC & BLACK PEPPER OATCAKES

A little turmeric goes a long way, as you'll see from the rich colour of these oatcakes.

---

250 g (8 oz) porridge oats
1 tablespoon olive oil
¼ teaspoon ground turmeric
good pinch of ground black pepper
¼ teaspoon sea salt flakes
flour, for dusting

Preheat the oven to 180°C (350°F), Gas Mark 4 and line a large baking tray with baking paper (parchment).

Put the oats into a large bowl. Add the olive oil, turmeric, pepper and sea salt and mix together.

Half fill a jug (pitcher) with boiled water and top it up with cool water. Add enough of it to the oats to make them form a ball that binds together. If you add too much water, just add some more oats.

Lightly flour a work surface and roll the ball into a large rectangle about 3 mm (¼ in) thick. Use a round cutter (about 6–7 cm/2½–3 in in diameter) to cut circles, then use a spatula to lift them on to the lined baking tray.

Bake until golden, 20–30 minutes, depending on thickness. Transfer to a wire rack to cool.

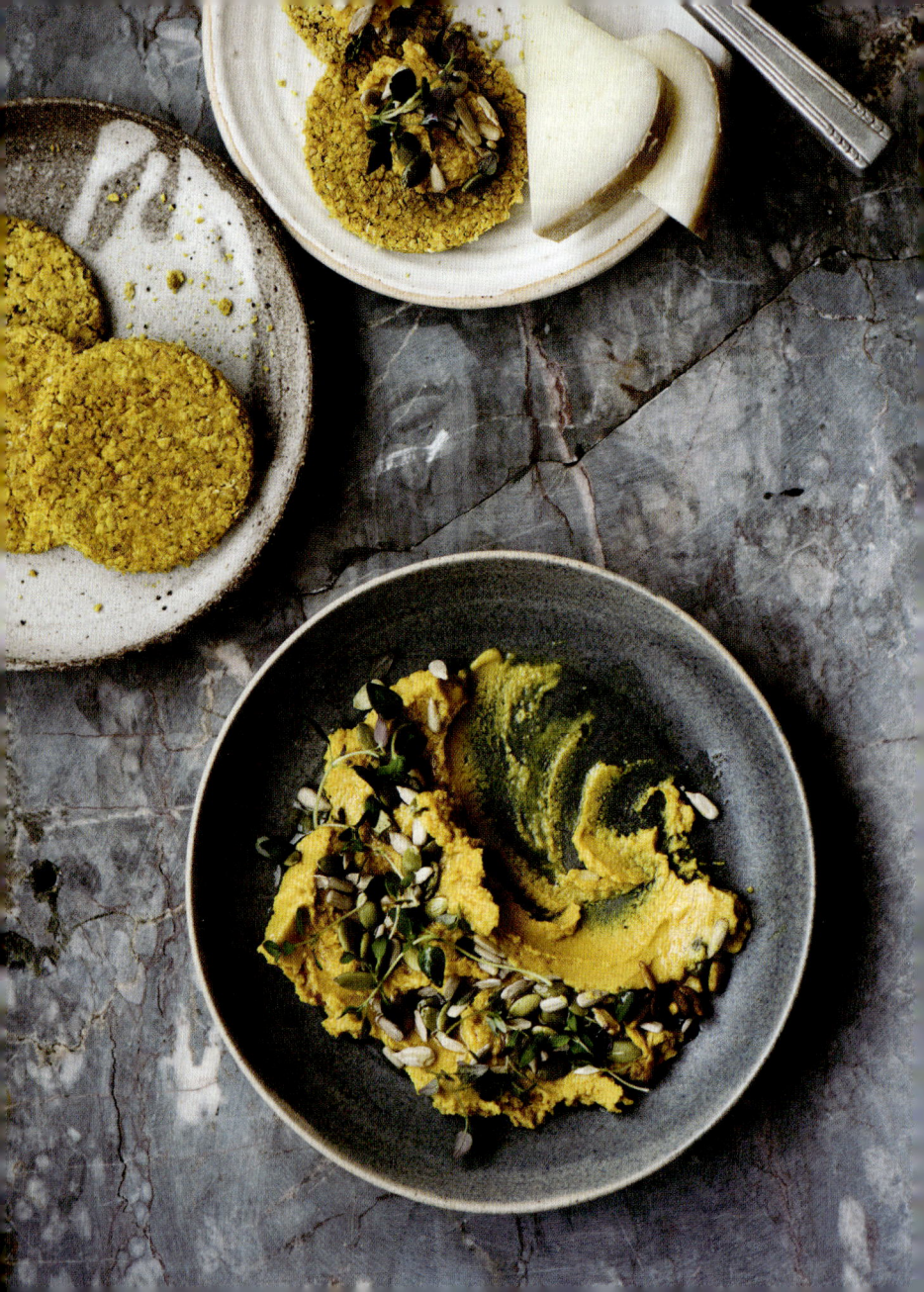

MAKES 400 G (13 OZ)

TURMERIC HUMMUS

For a cheat's version of this, simply stir a little ground turmeric and lemon zest into ready-made hummus, although there's something about making your own that can't be beaten.

---

400 g (13 oz) can chickpeas, rinsed and drained
zest and juice of 1 lemon
1 teaspoon sweet paprika
1 teaspoon ground turmeric
½ teaspoon mild chilli powder
6 tablespoons extra virgin olive oil, plus extra for drizzling
2 tablespoons tahini
1 teaspoon sea salt flakes
2 tablespoons water, plus more if needed

TO SERVE
honey or olive oil, for drizzling (optional)
spiced & roasted seeds (see page 30)
a handful of microherbs
turmeric & black pepper oatcakes (see page 31), (optional)

Put all the main ingredients in a food processor and blend until smooth, scraping down the sides of the processor as you go. Add more water if needed to get the right consistency.

Transfer to a bowl and add a drizzle of honey or olive oil. Garnish with a sprinkling of roasted seeds and a handful of microherbs. Serve with oatcakes, if you like.

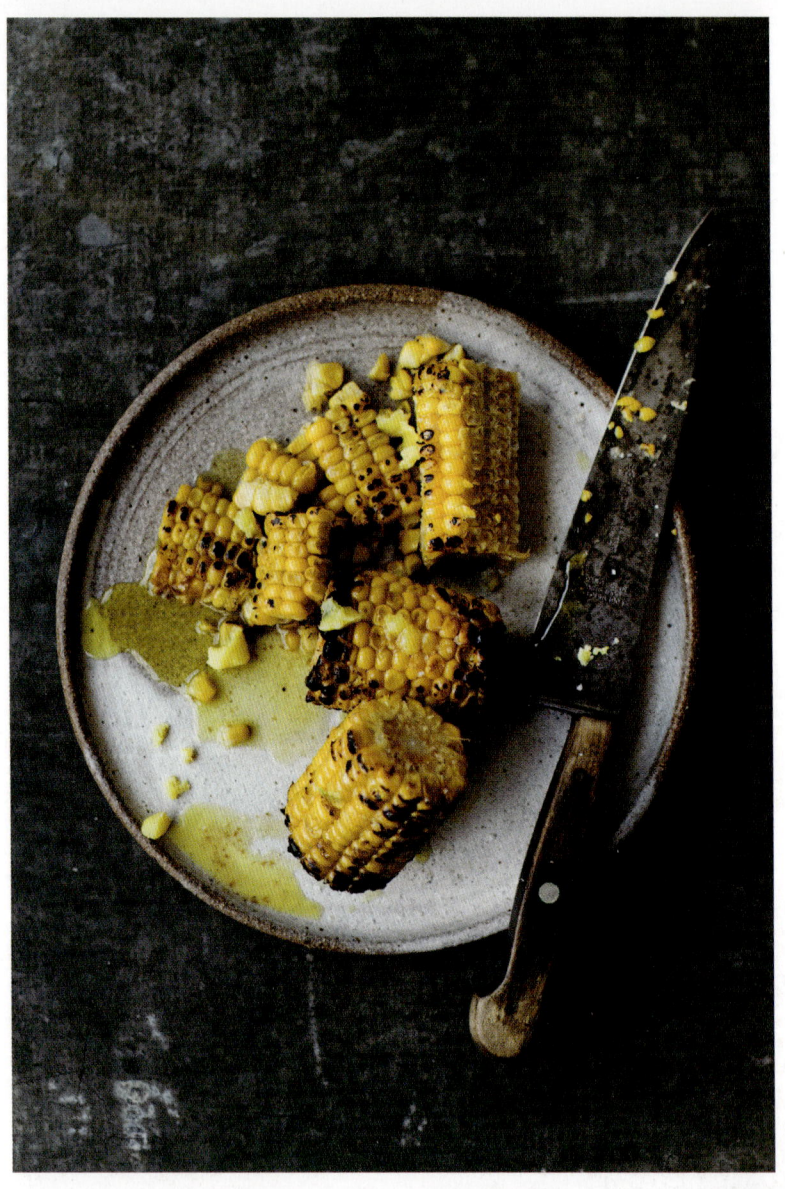

SERVES 4 AS A SIDE DISH

CORN ON THE COB
with turmeric butter

This is perfect for a summer barbecue. Adding spices to the butter gives an extra element of flavour. If you are using fresh corn on the cob, you will need to boil the pieces for about 10 minutes before grilling.

---

4 fresh or frozen corn cob pieces
80 g (3 oz) unsalted butter
½ teaspoon grated fresh turmeric or ground turmeric
½ teaspoon ground cumin
sea salt and ground black pepper

On a barbecue or in a hot griddle pan, cook the corn until soft and a little charred.

Melt the butter in a small saucepan and add the turmeric and cumin. Allow the spices to cook in the butter for a few minutes for the flavours to infuse.

Serve the corn with the melted butter poured over and season generously with salt and pepper.

SERVES 2

NEW POTATO SALAD
with turmeric tahini dressing

Potato salad is given a bit of a twist here, as the usual mayo is replaced with a vibrant tahini and turmeric dressing.

---

500 g (1 lb) new potatoes, washed
leaves from ½ bunch of fresh mint
4 spring onions (scallions), thinly sliced on the diagonal
1 teaspoon sumac
sea salt and ground black pepper

FOR THE DRESSING
80 g (3 oz) tahini
juice of 1 lemon
30 ml (1 fl oz) extra virgin olive oil
2 tablespoons water
1 teaspoon ground turmeric

Put the potatoes in a large pan and add enough cold water to cover them fully. Add a small handful of salt and 2 sprigs of the mint before covering with a lid. Place over a high heat and bring to the boil. Reduce the heat slightly and allow to simmer until the potatoes are easily pierced with a sharp knife.

Drain and allow to cool slightly – it's best to serve the salad warm but not piping hot.

In the meantime, make the dressing for the potatoes. Pour the tahini, lemon juice, olive oil, water and turmeric into a large bowl and whisk until smooth. If the dressing looks like the oil is separating, just whisk in a tablespoon of water at a time until the dressing is thick and glossy. Season with a generous pinch of salt and pepper.

Toss the warm potatoes in the dressing, add the remaining mint leaves and the spring onions and mix until thoroughly combined. Tip into a serving bowl and sprinkle the sumac evenly over the top.

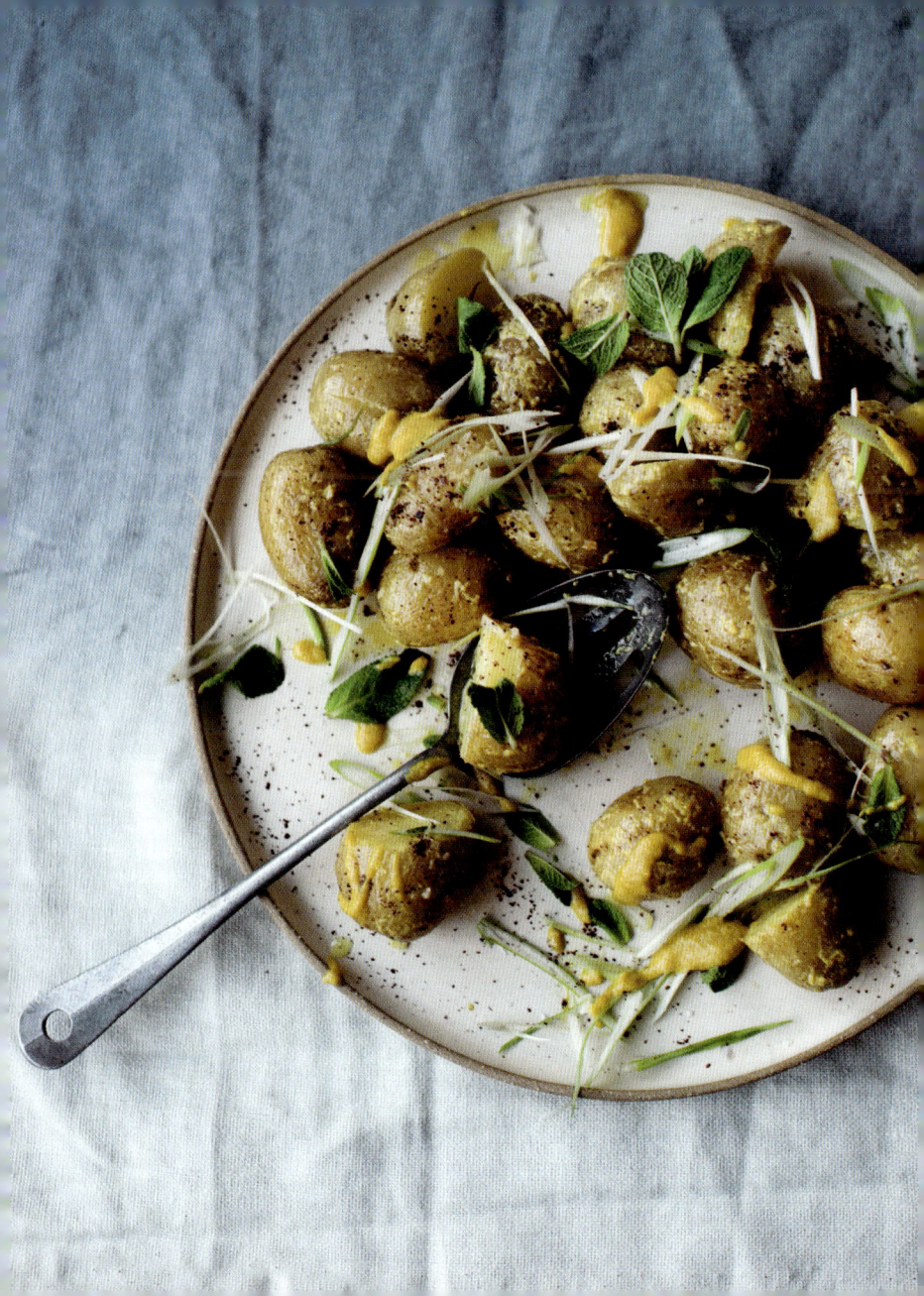

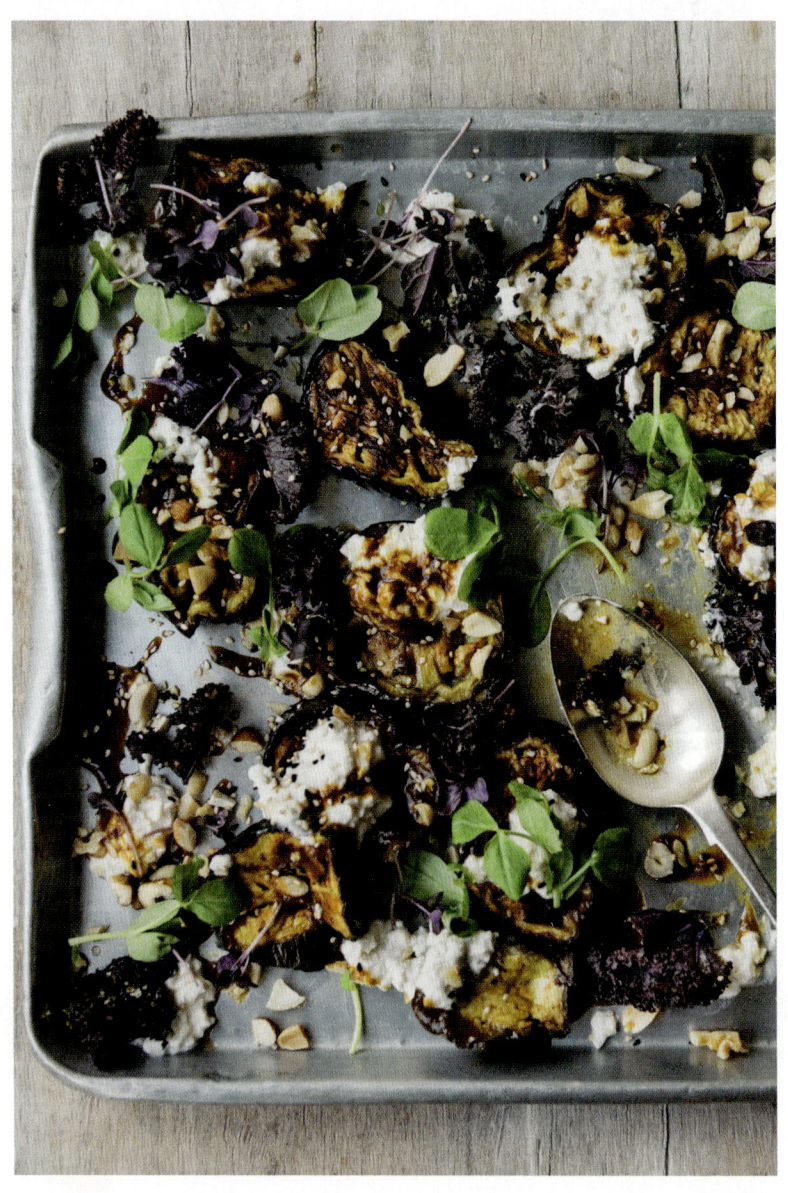

SERVES 4–6 AS A SIDE DISH

ROAST AUBERGINE
with tofu & turmeric dengaku

This is vegan heaven. Combining tofu and coconut milk creates a creamy dressing, while the miso turmeric dengaku glaze gives an umami flavour to the aubergine. It's a salad to impress friends with.

2–3 aubergines (depending on size), sliced into 2.5 cm (1 in) rounds
olive oil, for coating
1 tablespoon white miso
2 tablespoons cooking sake
1 teaspoon ground turmeric
1 tablespoon golden caster (light brown) sugar
100 g (3½ oz) kale, tough stems discarded and leaves roughly chopped
1 tablespoon soy sauce
1 teaspoon soft light brown sugar
200 g (7 oz) firm tofu
50 ml (2 fl oz) coconut milk
sea salt and ground black pepper

TO GARNISH
purple basil (optional)
2 tablespoons mixed chopped nuts
pea shoots

Preheat the oven to 230°C (450°F), Gas Mark 8.

Put the aubergine rounds in a large bowl and toss with plenty of olive oil and some sea salt. Arrange the rounds in a large roasting tray.

Whisk the miso, sake, turmeric and sugar together to make a loose paste. Brush over the aubergine slices and roast in the oven for about 10 minutes Turn them over, brush with the paste again and roast for another 10 minutes, until soft and deep golden in colour. Remove from the oven and allow to cool a little.

Meanwhile, toss the kale with the soy sauce and brown sugar and spread out on a baking tray. As soon as you have removed the aubergine, put the kale in the oven and switch it off to allow the kale to crisp in the residual heat while you arrange the salad.

Blitz the tofu and the coconut milk using either a food processor or a hand-held blender for just a few seconds to create a creamy, crumbly texture.

Arrange the aubergine rounds on a salad platter and sprinkle with the tofu and crispy kale. Garnish with some purple basil, if using, chopped nuts, a few pea shoots and a grinding of black pepper.

MAKES 1 LOAF

TURMERIC BANANA BREAD

This is a really easy and tasty way to use up overripe bananas. While spelt flour is used here, you could just as easily use a gluten-free flour. The coconut oil and bananas help to keep the loaf moist, and it's delicious toasted with a little butter.

---

200 g (7 oz) spelt flour
2 teaspoons baking powder
½ teaspoon bicarbonate of soda (baking soda)
¾ teaspoon sea salt
1 teaspoon ground ginger
1 teaspoon ground turmeric
50 ml (2 fl oz) coconut oil, melted
50 g (2 oz) coconut sugar or soft light brown sugar
1 teaspoon vanilla extract
3–4 ripe bananas, mashed
2 large eggs
butter, to serve

Preheat the oven to 180°C (350°F), Gas Mark 4 and oil or butter a 21 x 11 cm (8 x 4 in) loaf tin.

Sift the flour, baking powder, bicarbonate of soda, salt, ginger and turmeric into a bowl. In another bowl combine the melted coconut oil, coconut sugar, vanilla extract, mashed bananas and eggs until quite smooth, just with a few banana lumps.

Add the wet ingredients to the dry and stir until just combined into an airy batter. Scrape into the prepared loaf tin and bake until a skewer inserted in the centre comes out clean, about 50–60 minutes.

Allow to cool in the tin for 10 minutes, then run a knife around the edge of the loaf to release it; turn out on to a wire rack to cool completely. Cut into slices and serve, toasted if liked, and spread with butter. If stored in an air tight container, the loaf will keep for 3–4 days.

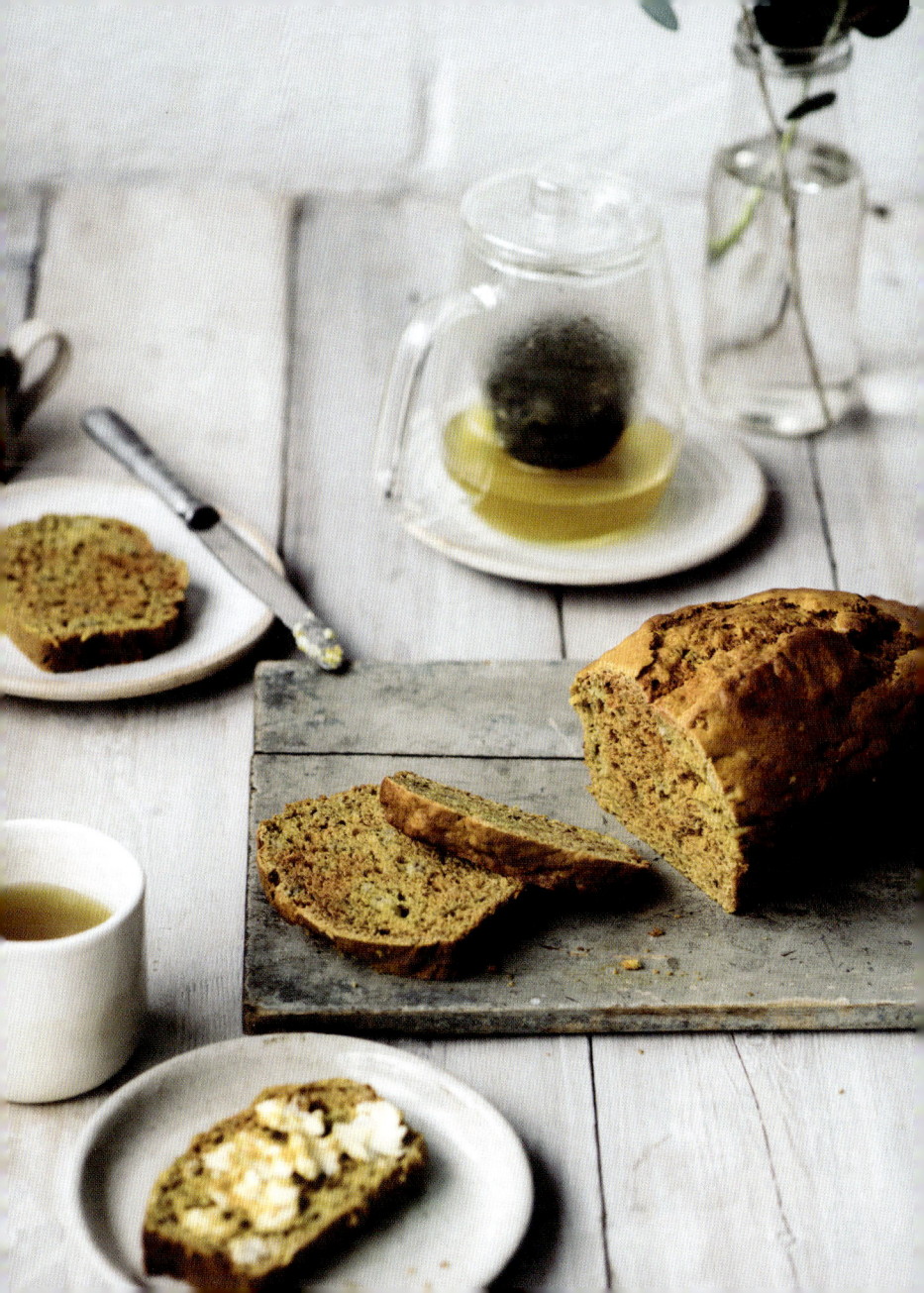

MAKES 3 × 200 G (7 OZ) JARS

TURMERIC PICKLES

Pickled vegetables have a pleasing sharpness and crunch, and are great for enjoying with a slice of cheese, cold cuts or on picnics.

---

200 g (7 oz) daikon radish, peeled
200 g (7 oz) carrots, peeled
200 g (7 oz) turnips
5 curry leaves per jar (fresh or dried)
1 red chilli per jar, deseeded and halved lengthways
2 strips of lemon rind per jar

FOR THE PICKLING LIQUOR
1.2 litres (2 pints) warm water
160 ml (5½ fl oz) rice wine vinegar
5 tablespoons coconut sugar or granulated sugar
2 tablespoons sea salt
½ teaspoon ground turmeric

Start by sterilizing the pickling jars you are going to use by pouring boiling-hot water into them and leaving them for several minutes. Pour the water out and leave them to air-dry.

Quarter the daikon radish lengthways so you have 4 long pieces, then cut each quarter into chunks. The carrots can be cut in half lengthways, then cut into chunky half-moons. You can cut the turnips any which way, as long as they are roughly the same size as the rest of the vegetables.

Divide them evenly between the jars but don't overpack them. Add the curry leaves, chillies and strips of lemon rind to the jars.

For the pickling liquor, heat the water and vinegar in a saucepan over a very low heat until it is nearly hot, then dissolve the sugar, salt and turmeric in it.

Pour the liquor evenly between the jars so the vegetables are covered. You may need to press the veg down slightly. Seal the jars and put in the refrigerator for 3 days to pickle. If you don't have 3 days to spare, you can bring the liquor to the boil before pouring it on to the veg, sealing the jar and allowing it to cool down. You don't get quite the full flavour but you will still have decent pickled veg.

MAKES 200 G (7 OZ)

TURMERIC MUSTARD

When you have a few pickles and condiments on hand, you'll be able to add the benefits of turmeric to your dishes without even thinking about it.

---

50 g (2 oz) mustard seeds (white or mixed)
25 g (1 oz) mustard powder
2 teaspoons sea salt flakes
150 ml (¼ fl oz) water
3 tablespoons apple cider vinegar
1 teaspoon ground turmeric
2 tablespoons raw clear (liquid) honey

Mix the mustard seeds, mustard powder and sea salt in a bowl, then add the water, combining well. Set aside for 10 minutes before adding the apple cider vinegar, turmeric and honey; mix well.

Transfer to an airtight jar and allow to set overnight in the refrigerator. The mustard will keep for up to 6 months in the refrigerator.

MAKES 500 ML (17 FL OZ)

TURMERIC-INFUSED OIL

When you have this oil on hand in the kitchen, you can make quick dressings or simply drizzle it over dishes both to add flavour and to give an immediate health boost.

---

250 ml (8 fl oz) avocado oil
250ml (8 fl oz) extra virgin olive oil
2 tablespoons grated fresh turmeric, or 2 heaped tablespoons ground turmeric
1 teaspoon coarsely ground black pepper

Add all the ingredients to a glass bottle, seal and shake. Leave to infuse for 2 weeks before using.

MAIN DISHES

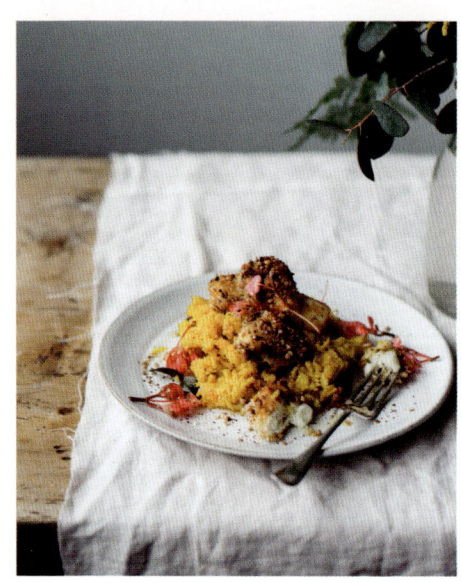

45	**Yellow Rice**
46	**Sweet Potato Bulgur**
47	**Five Veg Tagine**
49	**Roast Cauliflower Salad**
50	**Buddha Bowl**
52	**Bhindi Masala Curry**
53	**Turmeric Gnocchi**
55	**Turmeric Prawn Linguine**
56	**Miso Turmeric Glazed Salmon**
59	**Keralan Fish Curry**
60	**Turmeric & Tamarind Cod**
61	**Mussels**
62	**Beef Stew**
64	**Roast Chicken**

SERVES 2 (OR 4 AS A SIDE)

YELLOW RICE
with coconut halloumi

This coconut fried halloumi is a winner every time and is a very nice treat with a bowl of hot, steaming yellow rice.

---

zest of 1 lemon
1 teaspoon ground turmeric
1 teaspoon ground ginger
2 teaspoons yellow mustard seeds
150 g (5 oz) basmati rice, rinsed
300 ml (11 fl oz) hot vegetable stock (broth)
8 kaffir lime leaves
100 g (3½ oz) halloumi cheese, cubed
flour, for dusting
1 egg, beaten
50 g (2 oz) coconut flakes
vegetable oil, for frying
apple blossom flower, to garnish (optional), or use mint sprigs

Dry-fry the lemon zest, turmeric, ginger and yellow mustard seeds in a saucepan until the seeds begin to pop. Add the rice, stock and kaffir lime leaves and bring to the boil. Reduce the heat and simmer for 10 minutes, or until the rice is fluffy and cooked and all the liquid has been absorbed.

For the halloumi, dip the cubes first into some flour, then the beaten egg, and finally the coconut flakes, pressing to coat on all sides.

Heat a shallow depth of vegetable oil in a wok and fry the coconut halloumi cubes until golden brown on all sides. Carefully remove with a slotted spoon and drain on kitchen paper (paper towel).

Fluff up the rice with a fork and top with the fried halloumi. Garnish with apple blossom, if using, and serve immediately.

SERVES 2

SWEET POTATO BULGUR

Grain salads are a great choice for a lunchbox or sharing salad platter as the grain makes it feel more filling. You can mix and match your grains and roasted vegetables – for example, carrots with freekeh or butternut squash wedges with cracked wheat.

---

1 large sweet potato, roughly chopped
1½ teaspoons ground turmeric
1 teaspoon cumin seeds
2–3 tablespoons olive oil
100 g (3½ oz) bulgur wheat
1 teaspoon bouillon powder
100 g (3½ oz) baby spinach (shredded) or baby kale
2 tablespoons extra virgin olive oil
zest and juice of ½ lime
50 ml (2 oz) baked kefir or natural (plain) yogurt
sea salt
fresh coriander (cilantro) leaves, to serve

Preheat the oven to 220°C (425°F), Gas Mark 7.

Put the potatoes in a large bowl with 1 teaspoon of the ground turmeric, the cumin seeds, olive oil and a good pinch of salt and mix together. Transfer to a roasting tin and roast for about 20 minutes until the sweet potatoes are soft and a little crispy at the edges. Turn halfway through cooking.

Place the bulgur wheat in a saucepan, cover with 1 litre (1¾ pints) of water, then add the bouillon and remaining ground turmeric. Bring to the boil, then reduce the heat and simmer for 10–12 minutes, until cooked. Drain.

Toss the bulgur and roast sweet potato together with the spinach or kale and some extra virgin olive oil in a large bowl. Transfer to a salad platter.

Mix the lime zest and juice into the kefir or yogurt and drizzle over the salad, then scatter over the coriander leaves. Serve warm, or leave to cool, then chill in the refrigerator until needed.

SERVES 6

FIVE VEG TAGINE

While this recipe does have quite a long list of ingredients, the process is fairly simple and results in a great depth of flavour. Many of the spices are things that you can keep in your storecupboard, but feel free to mix and match along with the vegetables. This recipe works really well in big batches that you can keep in the refrigerator and then simply heat up later in the week.

½ tablespoon ground turmeric
½ tablespoon ground ginger
½ tablespoon dried chilli flakes
½ tablespoon ground cumin
½ tablespoon ground coriander
seeds from 4 cardamom pods
1 garlic clove, crushed
juice of 1 lemon
100 ml (3½ fl oz) olive oil
2 carrots, cut into wedges
½ butternut squash, peeled and cut into bite-sized pieces
2 small turnips, cut into wedges
½ celeriac (celery root), peeled and cut into bite-sized pieces
1 aubergine (eggplant), cut into 2 cm (¾ in) dice
400 g (13 oz) can chickpeas, rinsed and drained
500 ml (1 lb) vegetable stock (broth)
1 tablespoon tomato purée (paste)
sea salt and ground black pepper
couscous and natural yogurt, to serve

Preheat the oven to 200°C (400°F), Gas Mark 6.

Mix all the spices, garlic, lemon juice and olive oil in a bowl and season with salt and pepper. Add all the vegetables and mix thoroughly.

Place a large flameproof casserole dish over a medium heat, add the vegetables and let the mixture infuse for a few minutes. Now add the chickpeas, vegetable stock and tomato purée. Give everything a stir, cover and put in the oven for 30–40 minutes, until the vegetables are cooked and the flavours have all infused.

Prepare your couscous and spoon into bowls. Ladle the tagine over the couscous and serve with a spoonful of yogurt on top.

MAIN DISHES

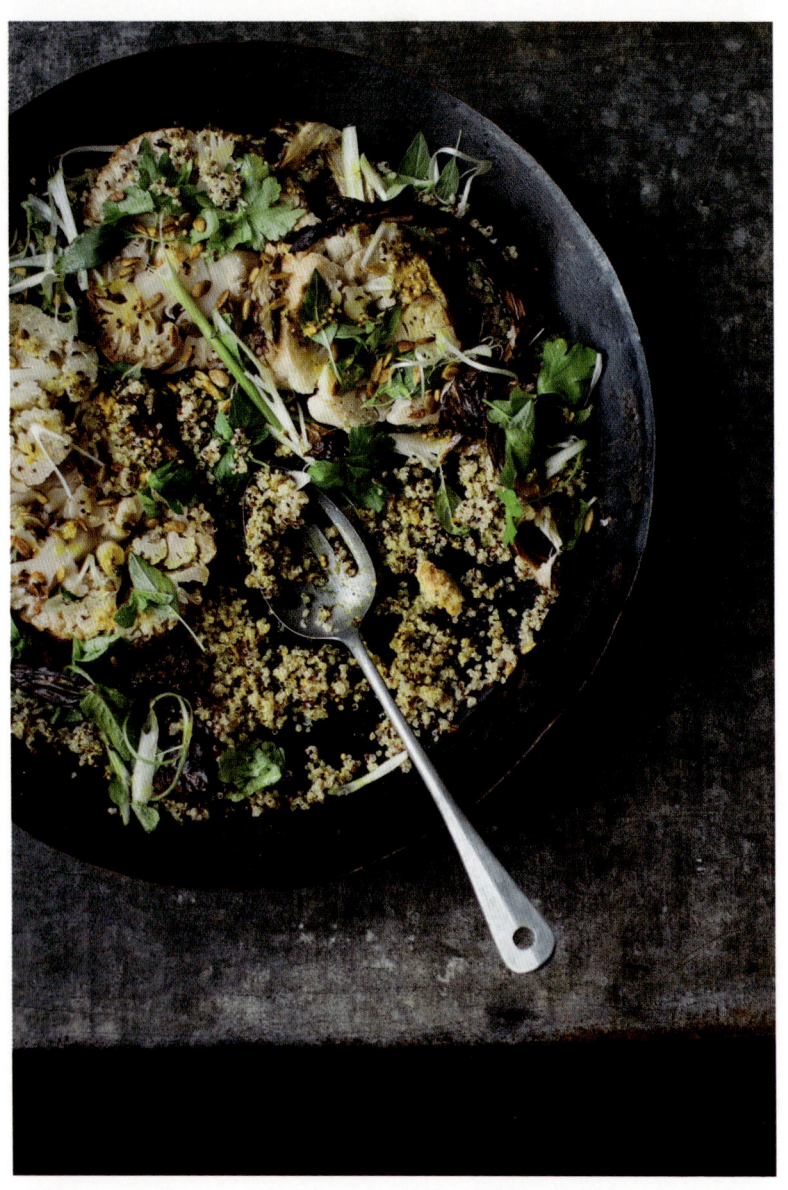

SERVES 4–6 AS A SIDE DISH

ROAST CAULIFLOWER SALAD
with ginger, turmeric & lime dressing

Roasting cauliflower whole is now a popular technique: it's a simple way to cook this versatile vegetable and gives it a lovely sweetness. The turmeric is in the dressing, which you toss the cauliflower in before serving with quinoa and spring onion and fresh coriander to finish.

---

1 medium cauliflower
4 tablespoons olive oil
1 teaspoon yellow mustard seeds
1 teaspoon fennel seeds
1 teaspoon ground coriander
1 teaspoon ground cumin
1 teaspoon ground turmeric
juice of 1 lime
5 cm (2 in) piece of fresh root ginger, peeled and grated
100 g (3½ oz) mixed quinoa
sea salt flakes

TO SERVE

3 spring onions (scallions), thinly sliced on the diagonal
handful of coriander (cilantro) leaves
handful of Thai basil leaves (optional)
spiced & roasted seeds (see page 30, optional)

Preheat the oven to 220°C (425°F), Gas Mark 7.

To roast the cauliflower whole, simply place on a roasting tray, drizzle over half the olive oil and sprinkle with sea salt. Roast for 45–60 minutes, or until the cauliflower is golden in colour and can be easily pierced with a sharp knife. Remove from the oven and allow to cool a little before slicing into thick 'steaks'.

Meanwhile, make the dressing. Heat the remaining oil in a saucepan and add the mustard seeds, stirring for about 1 minute over a medium–high heat until they begin to pop. Add the seeds and ground spices. Cook, stirring, for another minute or so, until fragrant. Remove the pan from heat and mix in the lime juice and ginger. Allow to cool and season with salt.

Mix the cauliflower in the dressing in a large bowl (don't worry if the cauliflower breaks up into florets) and leave to marinate while you cook the quinoa according to the packet instructions. Drain and set aside to cool.

Mix the quinoa into the dressed cauliflower and arrange on a salad platter. Scatter over the spring onions and fresh coriander, plus the Thai basil and spiced and roasted seeds, if using, just before serving.

SERVES 1

BUDDHA BOWL

The idea of the Buddha bowl is to have something plant-based from each of the main food groups – in other words, some protein, good carbohydrates, healthy fats and plenty of fresh veg. With this recipe you get all that goodness plus the added benefits of some turmeric thrown in. The trick here is to cook the individual elements of the bowl separately so that you can enjoy all the layers and flavours.

---

100 g (3½ oz) cooked Yellow Rice (see page 45) or cooked basmati rice

unsalted butter or coconut oil, for frying

1 roasted garlic clove (wrap a whole garlic bulb with sea salt in foil and roast in a low oven for 1 hour)

50 g (2 oz) mixed oriental mushrooms

1 tablespoon white wine

½ teaspoon harissa

50 g (2 oz) baby spinach

50 g (2 oz) green beans

1 teaspoon grated fresh turmeric or ground turmeric

25 g (1 oz) firm tofu

1 black radish, scrubbed and thinly sliced

½ teaspoon grated fresh root ginger or ground ginger

¼ Chinese cabbage, shredded

sea salt flakes

Cook the rice and keep warm in a low oven – around 150°C (300°F), Gas Mark 2.

Melt about 1 teaspoon butter or coconut oil in a hot frying pan (skillet) and squeeze in the roasted garlic clove. Stir for a few moments before adding the mushrooms, tossing continuously until golden and cooked. Deglaze the pan with the wine, transfer to a bowl and keep warm in the oven with the rice.

In the same pan, fry off the harissa. Add the baby spinach to wilt, then toss in the harissa. Set aside.

Heat a little coconut oil in a pan and add the green beans, turmeric and tofu, along with a little salt, scrambling the tofu as you cook the beans. Remove from the pan and set aside.

Finally, melt a little more butter or coconut oil in the pan, add the grated ginger and wilt the Chinese cabbage for a minute or two.

Assemble your bowl with all the elements and serve.

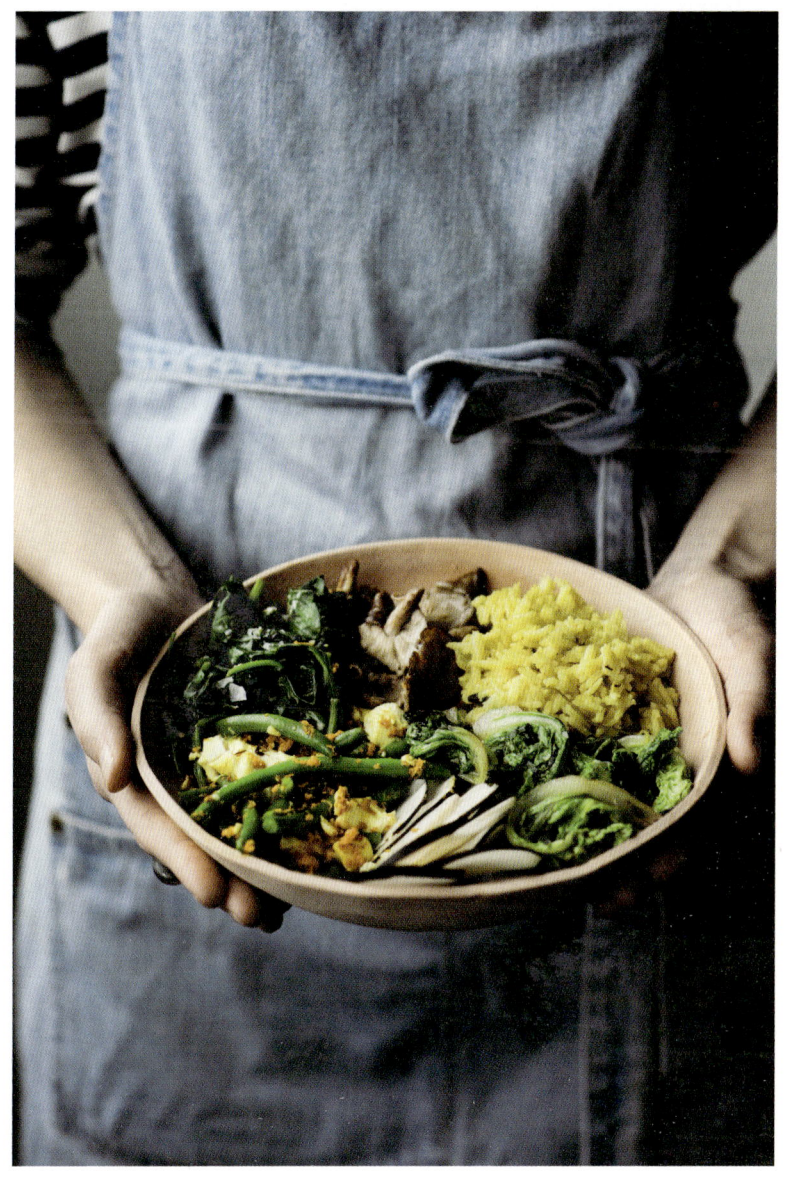

MAIN DISHES

SERVES 4 AS A SIDE DISH

BHINDI MASALA CURRY

This is a lightly spiced North Indian dish using the rather unheralded okra (bhindi), which you do have to be careful not to overcook or it becomes slimy. It's delicious in this traditional veg curry.

---

2 tablespoons coconut oil
300 g (10 oz) okra, each sliced at an angle into 3–4 pieces
1 large onion, finely diced
1 bay leaf
1 teaspoon ground turmeric
½ teaspoon chilli powder
½ teaspoon ground coriander
½ teaspoon ground cumin
200 ml (7 fl oz) water
10 g (⅓ oz) fresh coriander (cilantro), chopped
sea salt flakes
rice or Indian bread, to serve

FOR THE TOMATO PASTE

3 ripe tomatoes
1 cm (½ in) piece of fresh root ginger, peeled and roughly chopped
4 garlic cloves
2 green chillies
2 cloves
½ teaspoon ground cinnamon
2 tablespoons natural (plain) yogurt

First make the tomato paste: put the tomatoes, ginger, garlic and chillies in a food processor or blender and whizz together until completely smooth. Crush the cloves with the cinnamon and add to the paste. Stir in the yogurt and set aside.

Melt half the coconut oil in large frying pan (skillet) over a low heat and fry the okra for 10–15 minutes, until almost cooked – still firm but slightly browned all over. Remove from the pan and drain on kitchen paper (paper towel).

In the same pan, add the remaining coconut oil and fry the onion with the bay leaf until completely soft and slightly caramelized. Add the ground spices and stir quickly so as not to burn them. Stir in the tomato paste and keep cooking over a low heat until the sauce has thickened. Add the water, season with salt and give it a very good stir. Return the okra to the sauce and cook for another 5 minutes. Do not cook for longer otherwise the okra will become extremely slimy.

Add the chopped coriander and serve with rice or a good Indian bread to soak up the sauce.

SERVES 4

TURMERIC GNOCCHI

Seaweed and turmeric make a surprisingly good combination. You don't need to go to all the trouble of making your own gnocchi to make this recipe, but you will notice the difference if you have the time and patience to give it a try.

---

4 large floury potatoes, such as Russet or Desirée
150 g (5 oz) plain flour, plus extra for dusting
2 teaspoons sea salt flakes
1 egg, beaten
100 g (3½ oz) unsalted butter, at room temperature, cut into small cubes
½ teaspoon ground turmeric
1 teaspoon nori or dulse seaweed flakes
1 tablespoon vegetable oil
50 g (2 oz) pecorino cheese, or any hard cheese, grated
handful of fresh chives, chopped
2 tablespoons spiced & roasted seeds (see page 30) or toasted pumpkin seeds
pea shoots, to garnish
ground black pepper

Preheat the oven to 220°C (425°F), Gas Mark 7.

Bake the potatoes for about 45 minutes, or until easily pierced with a sharp knife. When just cool enough to handle, peel the potatoes and pass through a potato ricer into a bowl. (Alternatively, mash until smooth, then push the mixture through a sieve.) Allow to cool.

Sift the flour into the potatoes and sprinkle with the salt. Create a small well in the middle and add the beaten egg. Stir together before tipping on to a floured surface. Knead the mixture until it is soft and smooth, then divide into 8 equal pieces. Roll these into long sausage ropes and cut into pieces about 2cm (¾ in) square.

Bring a saucepan of salted water to the boil and cook the gnocchi in batches – they are ready when they float to the surface, usually after a few minutes. Remove with a slotted spoon and drain on kitchen paper (paper towel).

When the gnocchi are cooked, melt the butter in a large frying pan (skillet) and add the turmeric and seaweed flakes. In a separate pan, heat the vegetable oil and fry the gnocchi. Divide among 4 bowls. Drizzle the flavoured butter and scatter with grated cheese, chives and toasted seeds. Finish with a few pea shoots and a grinding of black pepper. Serve immediately.

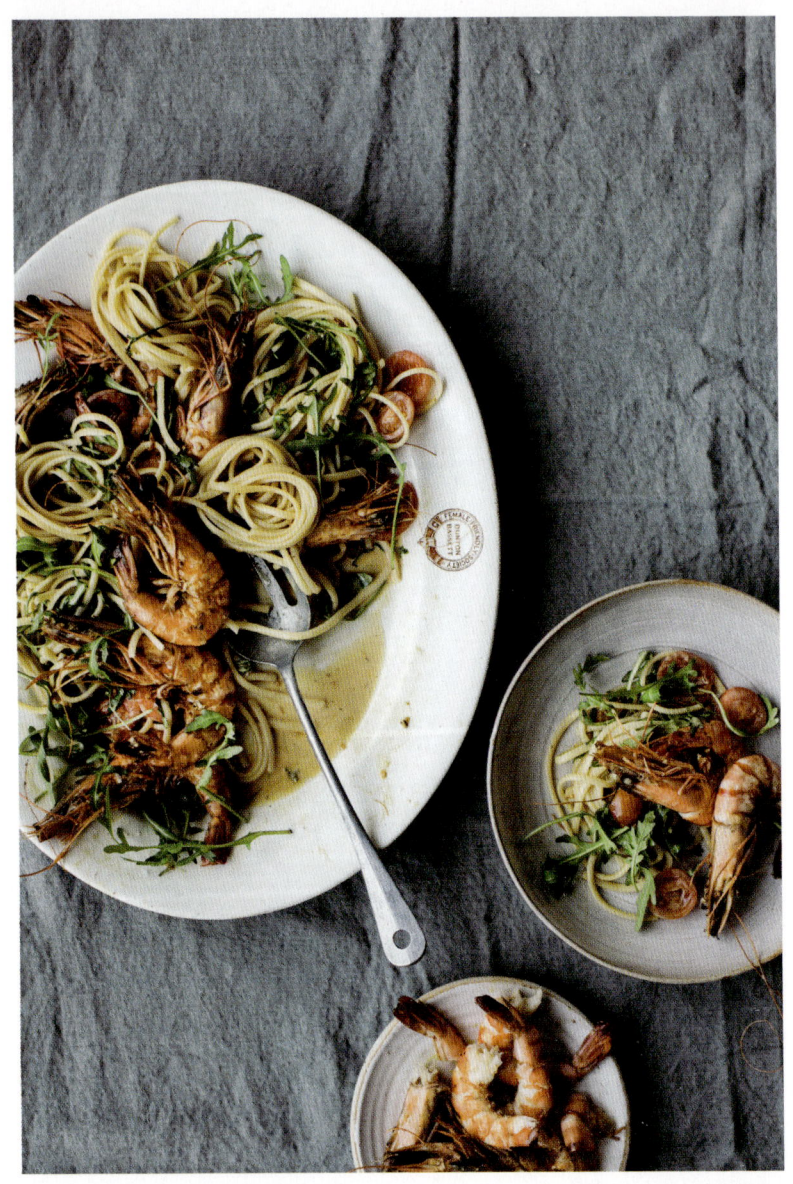

SERVES 2

TURMERIC PRAWN LINGUINE

This is a wonderful sharing dish. The traditional Mediterranean flavours work really well with the addition of turmeric and a fresh yogurt sauce.

---

2 tablespoons olive oil, plus extra for drizzling
½ shallot, finely diced
1 garlic clove, grated or very finely chopped
2.5 cm (1 in) piece of fresh root ginger, peeled and grated
1 teaspoon ground turmeric
200 g (7 oz) raw prawns (shrimp, ideally shell-on)
200 g (7 oz) linguine
150 g (5 oz) natural (plain) yogurt
50 g (2 oz) rocket (arugula)
8 cherry tomatoes, halved
sea salt and ground black pepper

Bring a large saucepan of salted water to the boil.

Meanwhile, heat the oil in a frying pan (skillet) over a low–medium heat. Add the shallot and fry gently until it becomes transparent. Add the garlic and ginger and continue to fry over a low heat for 4–5 minutes, until they are aromatic and soft. Add the turmeric and cook for another couple of minutes.

Increase the heat and add the prawns, stirring to coat them in the other ingredients. Cook for 4–8 minutes.

By this time, the water should be boiling, so add the linguine and cook according to the packet instructions. Drain the pasta, reserving a cupful of the water, and stir a little oil through it.

Once the prawns feel firm to touch and are pink all over, add the yogurt and half a ladleful of reserved pasta water. Cook, stirring, for 3–4 minutes to fully soak up the flavours, adding more water if necessary.

Season to taste and reduce the heat to very low. Add the drained pasta, rocket and tomatoes and stir through until the leaves have wilted. The pasta will soak up the sauce, so if it looks a little dry, add some more pasta water until you have a sauce that coats every strand. Serve immediately.

SERVES 2

MISO TURMERIC GLAZED SALMON
with wilted greens

The glaze for the salmon lifts this simple and healthy weeknight dinner to create something special. Salmon is full of healthy omega oils, which have a very important role in maintaining cells in the body.

---

1 tablespoon light sesame oil
2 x 150 g (5 oz) skin-on salmon fillets
1 tablespoon unsalted butter
½ teaspoon ground turmeric
pinch of ground black pepper
1 pak choi, leaves separated
100 g (3½ oz) mangetout (snow peas)
100 g (3½ oz) cavolo nero, stalks removed and leaves chopped
few slices of sushi ginger
2 tablespoons soy sauce

FOR THE GLAZE

2 tablespoons mirin
1 teaspoon coconut sugar, or use brown sugar (soft light)
1 garlic clove, roasted (see page 50)
1 teaspoon brown miso paste
1 teaspoon Turmeric Honey (see page 11, or use clear, liquid honey)

First make the glaze: put the mirin, sugar, garlic, miso paste and honey in a bowl and whisk together. Set aside.

Preheat the grill (broiler) to high. Place a nonstick frying pan (skillet) over a medium–high heat, add the sesame oil and fry the salmon, skin-side down, until the skin is golden and crisp. Turn over, brush with the miso turmeric glaze and place the pan under the grill for a few minutes.

Heat another large frying pan or wok over a high heat and add the butter, turmeric and black pepper. Add the pak choi, mangetout and cavolo nero. Toss for about 30 seconds, then add the sushi ginger and soy sauce.

When the greens are wilted, divide between 2 plates and top with the glazed salmon.

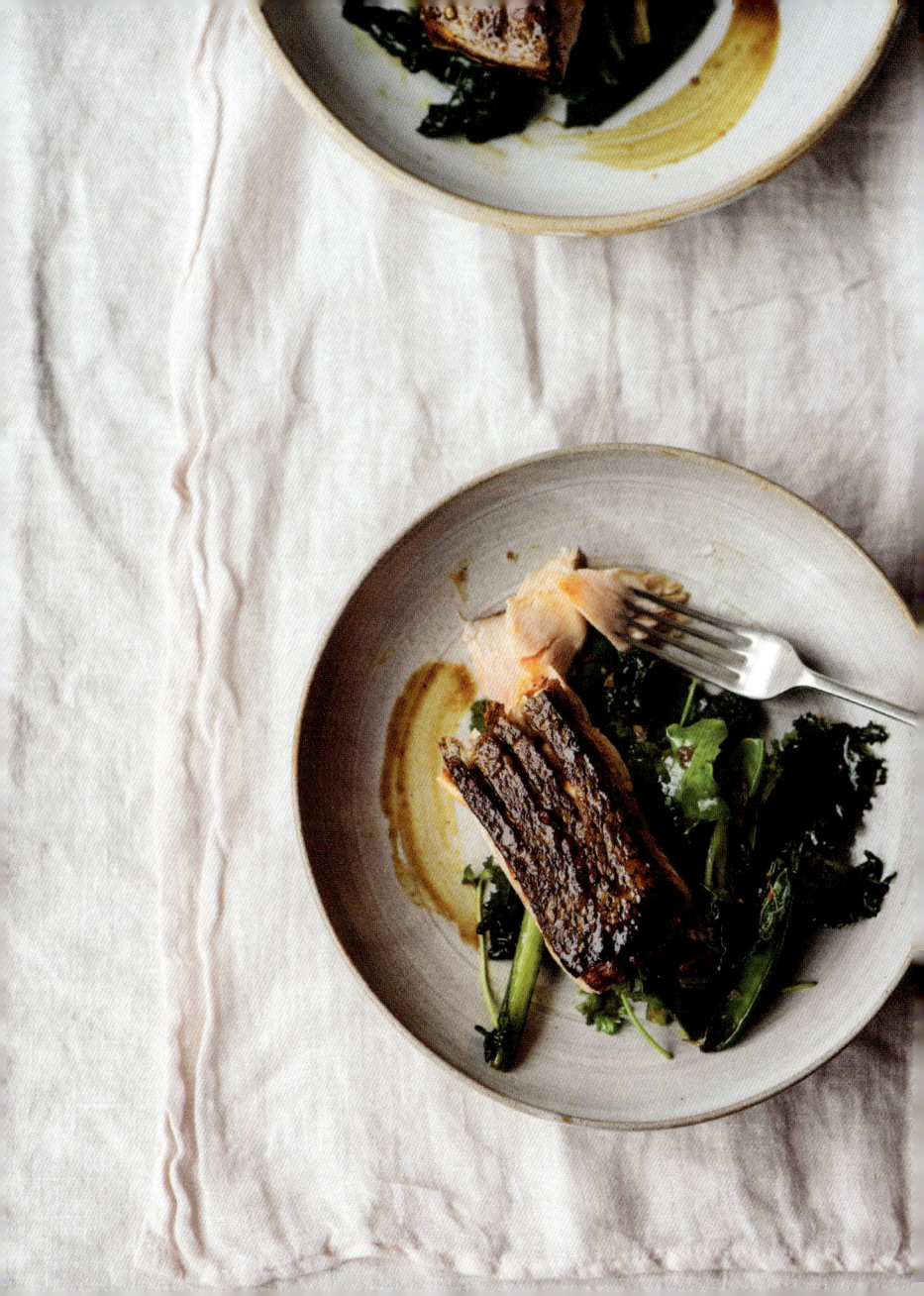

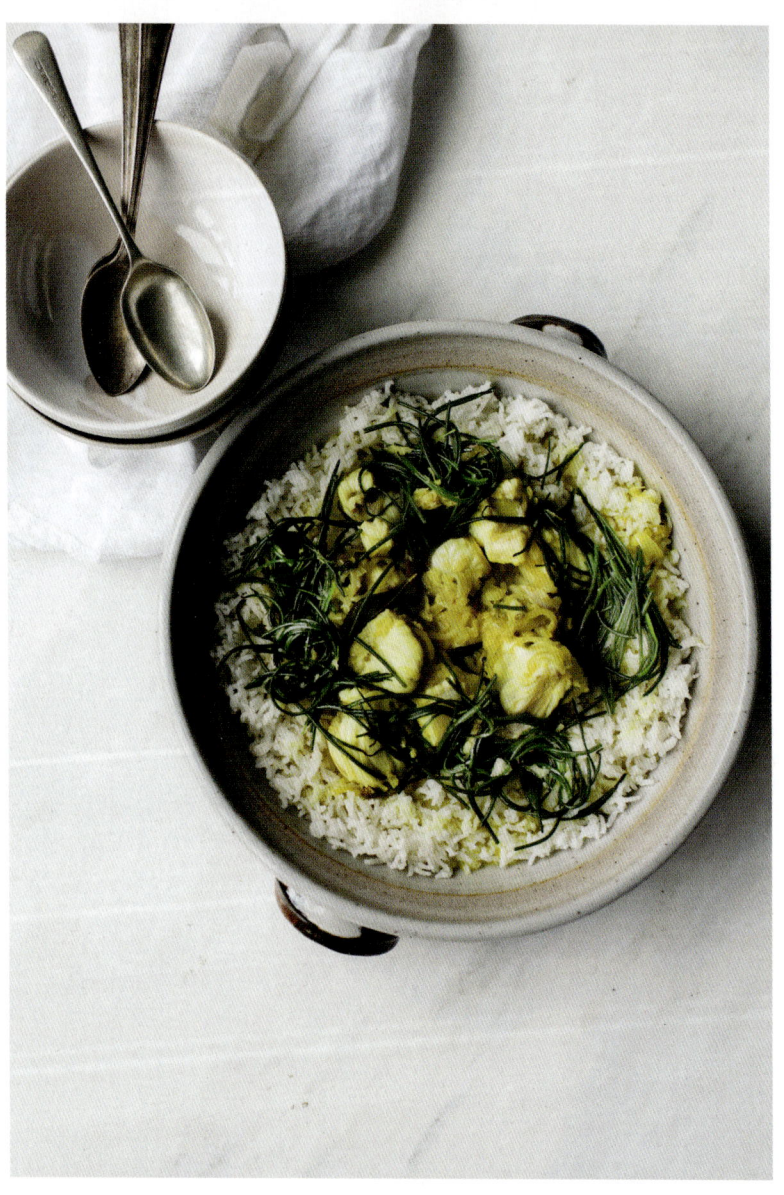

SERVES 2

KERALAN FISH CURRY

With its gentle combination of spices, this is a warming curry from the Ayurvedic tradition, balanced by coconut milk and lemon. It's a lovely fresh dish and you can use any firm, white-fleshed fish that is in season.

---

1 tablespoon groundnut oil
2.5 cm (1 in) piece of cinnamon stick
3 cloves
1/3 teaspoon mustard seeds
1/3 teaspoon fennel seeds
5 black peppercorns
½ onion, thinly sliced
7 dried curry leaves
150 g (5 oz) basmati rice
1½ teaspoons garlic paste
1½ teaspoons ginger paste
¼ teaspoon ground turmeric
pinch of sea salt
100 ml (3½ fl oz) water
100 ml (3½ fl oz) coconut milk
squeeze of lemon juice
250 g (8 oz) firm monkfish or cod, cut into large cubes
1 teaspoon unsalted butter or coconut oil
80 g (3 oz) monk's beard, samphire or baby spinach

Heat the oil in a large nonstick saucepan, add the whole spices and cook over a medium heat until the mustard seeds start popping. Add the onion and curry leaves and cook for a few minutes, until soft and translucent.

Meanwhile, cook the rice according to the packet instructions.

Add the garlic and ginger pastes to the spices and stir for a minute. Add the turmeric, salt and water. Bring to the boil, then reduce the heat and simmer for about 7 minute, until nicely reduced. Add the coconut milk, bring back to the boil and cook for a couple of minutes.

Squeeze in the lemon juice and add the fish in one layer, just covering it with the sauce. Simmer gently until the fish is cooked through, about 8 minutes (depending on the thickness of the fish). Taste for seasoning.

Heat the butter or coconut oil in a pan and sauté the monk's beard or samphire for a minute or two.

Serve the curry on the rice, with greens scattered over the top.

SERVES 2

TURMERIC & TAMARIND COD

This recipe marries turmeric with cod plus the honey in the salad dressing. The salad is raw, giving freshness and crunch to complement the gently cooked fish.

---

1 tablespoon tamarind paste
½ teaspoon grated fresh turmeric or ground turmeric
1 tablespoon hot water
2 x 200 g (7 oz) skin-on cod fillet pieces (ask the fishmonger to remove any bones)
½ onion, grated
good splash of rose or jasmine tea
lime wedges, to serve

FOR THE SALAD
½ white cabbage, finely chopped or grated
½ small cucumber (ideally Lebanese), sliced
½ red onion, thinly sliced
handful of any soft fresh herbs, such as basil, mint, dill
1 teaspoon black onion seeds
2 teaspoons manuka honey or raw honey
3 tablespoons natural (plain) yogurt
sea salt and ground black pepper

Mix the tamarind paste, turmeric and hot water in a large bowl until combined, then set aside to cool. Toss the fish in this marinade, then add the grated onion and chill in the refrigerator for 20 minutes.

Toss all of the salad ingredients together in a bowl until well combined. Season with salt and pepper and set aside.

Get a nonstick frying pan (skillet) really hot, then place the cod skin-side in it. Cook for 3 minutes, then turn the fish over and add a splash of tea. After the initial whoosh of the tea hitting the pan, reduce the heat, cover the pan and steam for about 5 minutes.

Pile the salad onto plates and top with the fish. Serve with lime wedges alongside for squeezing.

SERVES 4

MUSSELS
with turmeric & lemon grass

Mussels are wonderful for sharing and so simple to cook. They can take on lots of strong flavours, in this case the combination of turmeric, chilli and lemon grass, which works beautifully.

---

2 tablespoons coconut oil
4 garlic cloves, sliced
2 red chillies, deseeded and thinly sliced
1 lemon grass stalk, crushed along the stem and halved
½ teaspoon ground turmeric
1 kg (2 lb) fresh mussels, cleaned and beards removed
400 g (13 oz) cherry tomatoes, halved
1 bunch of fresh Thai basil, or use red basil or regular basil
sea salt and ground black pepper

Heat the coconut oil in a large, wide saucepan over a low–medium heat and add the garlic, chillies and lemon grass. Fry for a few minutes until they are aromatic and the garlic begins to brown slightly. Add the turmeric and cook for another 30 seconds.

Increase the heat to high and add the mussels and tomatoes. Season with salt and pepper, stir all together and cover the pan. Shake every now and again so the mussels are nudged open – this should take around 4–5 minutes.

Give the last few mussels a chance to open if they haven't already, but if any remain firmly shut, make sure you discard them before serving. When they're all opened you should have a lovely broth at the bottom made from the mussel and tomato juices.

Serve on a large sharing platter with plenty of Thai basil scattered over.

SERVES 4

BEEF STEW

Adding turmeric to stews is a simple way of incorporating a little more of this healthy spice into your cooking. With the ginger, it adds a touch of warmth to this hearty beef stew. Feel free to use any seasonal root veg and tubers you have to hand, such as parsnips, squash, swede (rutabaga) and celeriac (celery root).

---

olive oil, for frying
2 onions, sliced
400 g (13 oz) stewing steak, cut into chunks and seasoned with salt and pepper
1 teaspoon ground turmeric
1 teaspoon ground ginger
6 shallots, halved
12 baby carrots
8 baby turnips
1 litre (1¾ pints) vegetable stock (broth), or enough to cover the meat
Parmesan cheese rind (if you have one)
hunks of sourdough bread, to serve

Preheat the oven to 150°C (300°F), Gas Mark 2.

Heat a little olive oil in a large flameproof casserole dish and add the onions. Gently fry over a low–medium heat until softened. Set aside on a plate, then add a little more oil to the pan and start browning the steak in batches.

Return all the meat and the onions to the pan, add the turmeric and ginger, then cook slowly for 10 minutes.

Add the shallots, carrots, turnips, vegetable stock and Parmesan rind, if using. Cover and place in the oven for 3 hours. Check on it occasionally to make sure there is enough liquid to cover the meat and vegetables. If at any time it looks dry, top it up with more stock or a little water.

Serve with hunks of crusty sourdough bread to mop up the flavoursome juices.

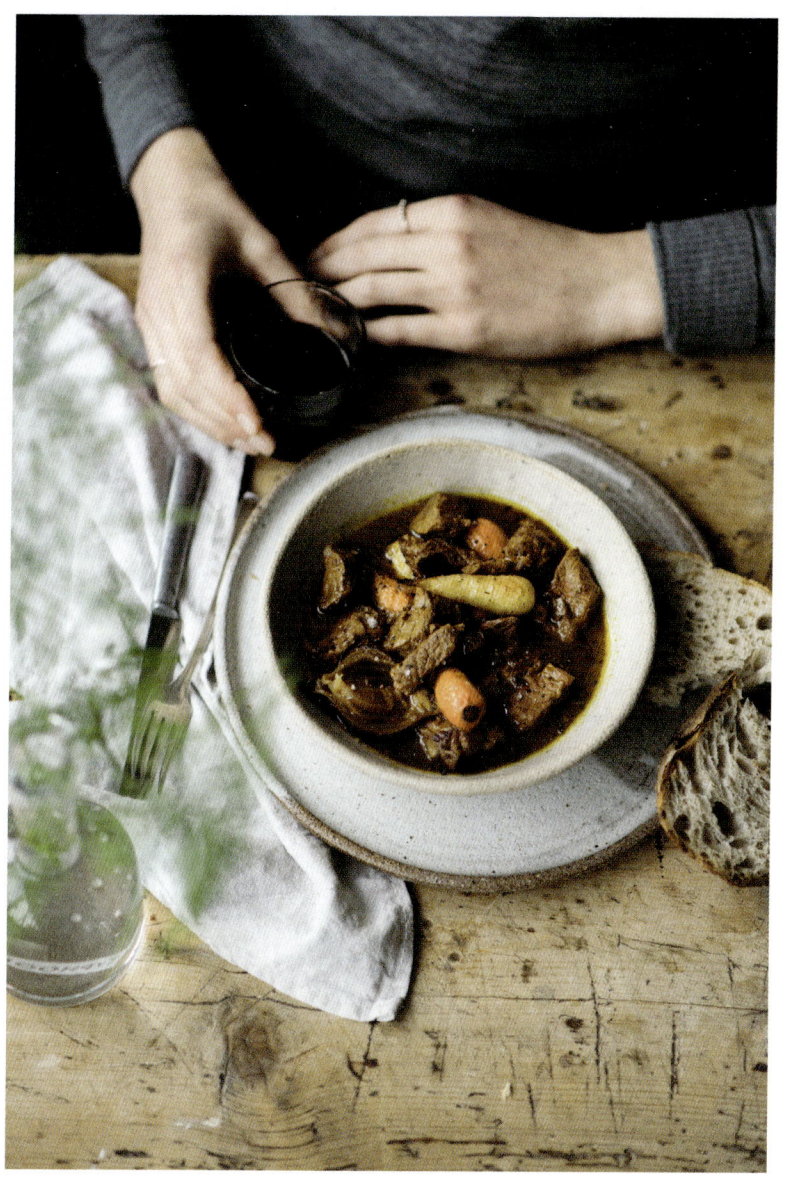

MAIN DISHES

SERVES 4

ROAST CHICKEN
with tandoori rub

The spices in this rub result in a subtle flavour that is not too heavy or overpowering, so this is definitely one to try for the next time you want to roast a whole chicken. You can skip the brining step if you are cooking on the day.

---

1 large whole chicken
1 lemon
400 g (13 oz) purple sprouting broccoli
olive oil, for drizzling
½ teaspoon dried chilli flakes
100 g (3½ oz) baby kale or baby leaf salad
sea salt flakes

FOR THE BRINE (OPTIONAL)
4.5 litres (9½ pints) cold water
85 g (3 oz) fine salt
200 g (7 oz) soft light brown sugar

FOR THE TANDOORI PASTE
2 tablespoons coconut oil
½ teaspoon ground ginger
1 teaspoon ground cumin
1 teaspoon garam masala
½ teaspoon chilli powder
½ teaspoon ground coriander
1 teaspoon ground turmeric
½ teaspoon ground black pepper
3 garlic cloves, crushed

If brining the chicken, start by whisking all the brine ingredients together until dissolved. Put the chicken into a stockpot or container big enough to hold it comfortably and pour over enough of the brine to cover it entirely. Leave for at least 3 hours but ideally overnight. Remove the chicken from the brine, rinse and pat dry with kitchen paper (paper towel).

Preheat the oven to 200°C (400°F), Gas Mark 6.

Pound or blend all the paste ingredients together so you have a thick rub. Slice the lemon into quarters and rub all over the chicken, inside and out. Now rub the paste all over, making sure you don't neglect the legs, thighs and wings.

Put the lemon quarters into the cavity, place the chicken in a roasting tray and cover with foil. Roast in the oven for 2 hours, then remove the foil, increase the heat to 240°C (475°F), Gas Mark 9 and cook for another 20 minutes, or until well browned. Remove from the oven and set aside to rest.

Steam the broccoli until al dente. Place in a bowl with the kale and toss with a little olive oil, the chilli flakes and some sea salt. Serve with the chicken.

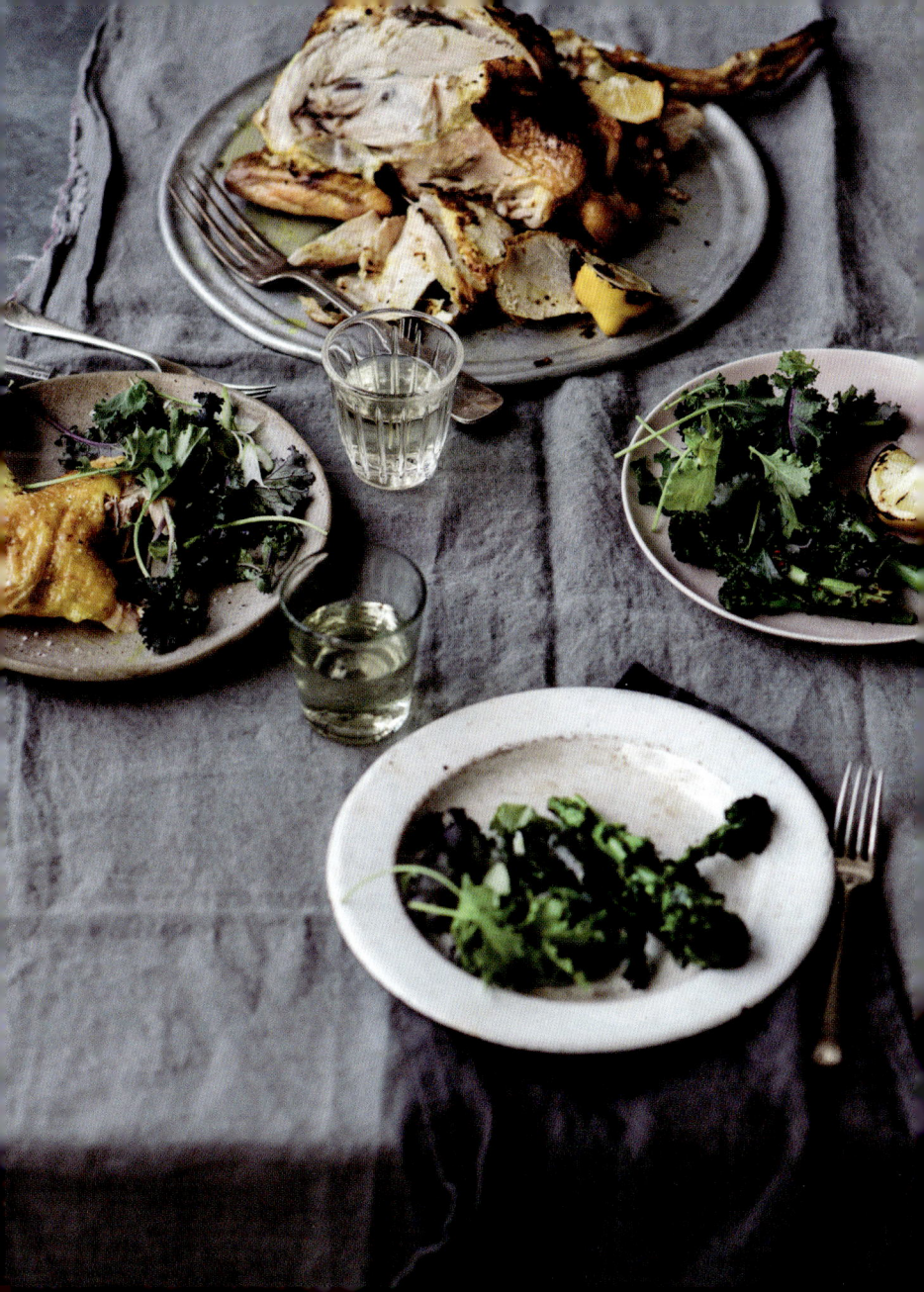

SWEETS & DRINKS

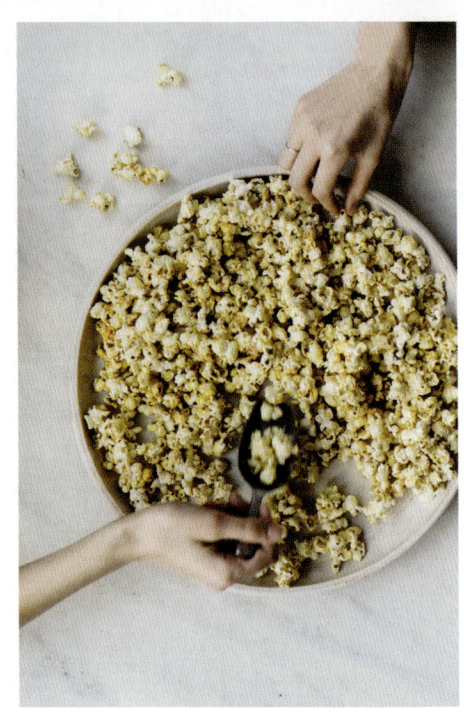

67	**Popcorn**
69	**Turmeric Maple Ice Cream**
70	**Turmeric Chai Muffins**
72	**Turmeric-Glazed Banana**
73	**Coconut Rice Pudding**
75	**Apple Turmeric Tonic**
75	**Turmeric Toddy**
76	**Turmeric Tea**
76	**Golden Mylk**

MAKES 1 BIG BOWL

POPCORN

This is such a simple but popular snack. If you prefer savoury to sweet, just replace the maple syrup with ½ teaspoon ground cumin.

---

2 tablespoons coconut oil
200 g (7 oz) popcorn kernels
½ teaspoon ground turmeric
¼ teaspoon dried chilli flakes
1 teaspoon sea salt flakes, or to taste
2 tablespoons maple syrup

Place a large, deep saucepan over a high heat. When the pan is hot, add the coconut oil and after about 30 seconds add the popcorn kernels.

Cover the pan and shake so that the kernels are all getting the heat as they pop. It's a bit tricky to know when all the kernels have popped if you don't have a glass lid, but when the popping noise stops for a few seconds, have a look.

Tip into a bowl and sprinkle over the turmeric, dried chilli flakes and sea salt. Drizzle over the maple syrup and shake until the seasoning is evenly distributed. Serve immediately.

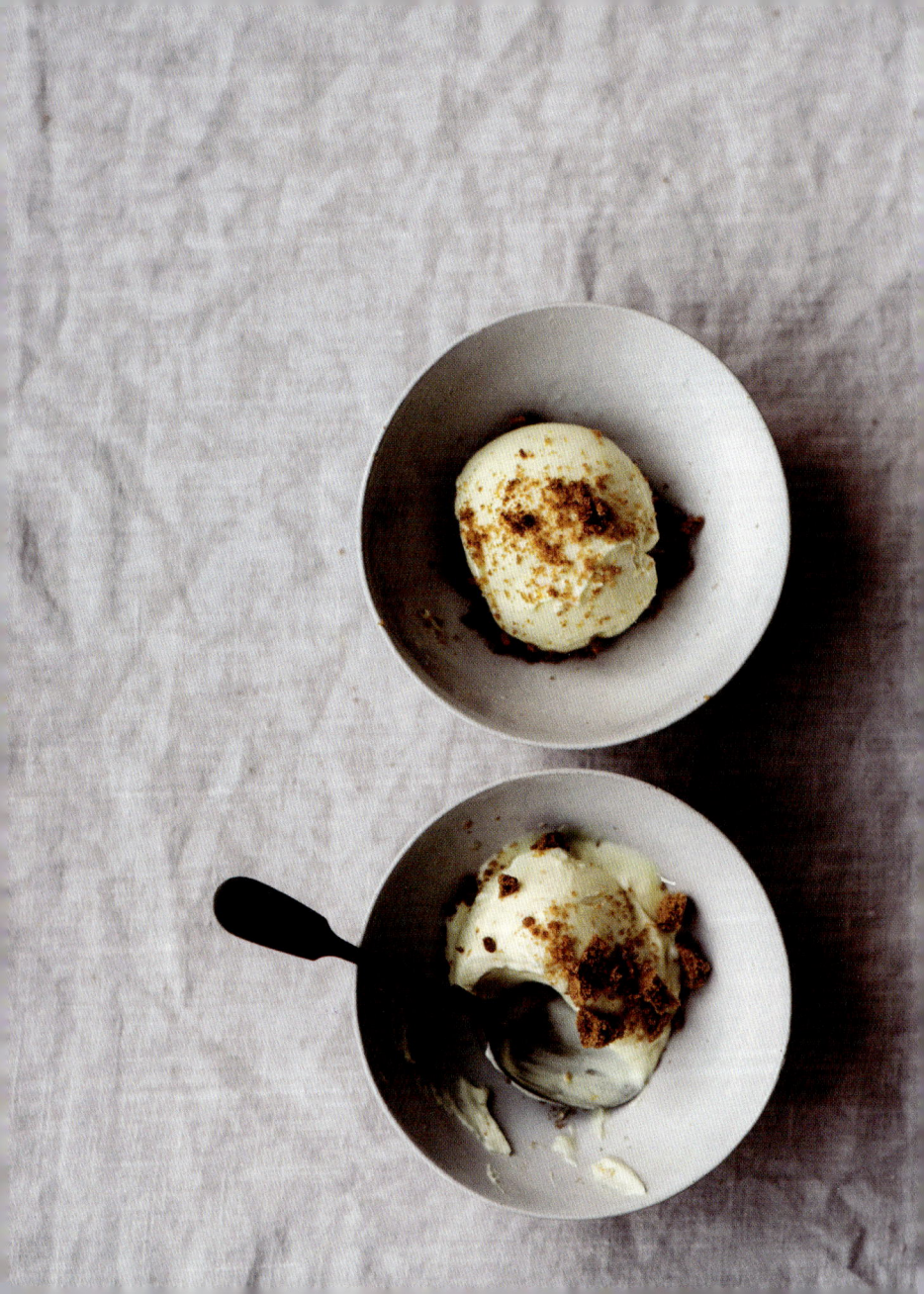

MAKES 1 LITRE (1¾ PINTS)

TURMERIC MAPLE ICE CREAM

You don't need an ice cream machine to make this recipe. If you do have a machine, you can use your favourite base recipe and add the maple syrup and turmeric to flavour your ice cream. It's surprising but the turmeric really works with the cream.

---

30 g (1 oz) maple syrup
1 teaspoon ground turmeric
600 ml (1 pint) double (heavy) cream
400 g (13 oz) can condensed milk
4 caramelized biscuits (such as Lotus Biscoff), crushed into fine crumbs

Gently heat the maple syrup and turmeric together in a small saucepan for a few minutes, just to infuse the flavours. Set aside to cool.

Put the cream and condensed milk into a large bowl and, using a hand-held electric whisk, beat for around 5 minutes or so until the mixture forms soft peaks.

Whisk the turmeric-infused maple syrup into the cream mixture, then spoon into a rigid freezerproof container.

Freeze overnight until the mixture is firm. Transfer to the refrigerator for 15–20 minutes before scooping. Serve the ice cream with the biscuit crumbs scattered over it.

MAKES 8 MUFFINS

TURMERIC CHAI MUFFINS

These muffins aren't particularly sweet and have a lovely soft texture, making them perfect for a weekend treat.

---

50 g (2 oz) unsalted butter, softened
120 g (4 oz) golden caster sugar
1 egg
½ teaspoon vanilla extract
175 g (6 oz) plain (all-purpose) flour
½ teaspoon salt
¾ teaspoon baking powder
¼ teaspoon bicarbonate of soda (baking soda)
1 teaspoon ground cinnamon
½ teaspoon ground turmeric
½ teaspoon ground ginger
½ teaspoon ground cardamom
¼ teaspoon ground black pepper
100 ml (3½ fl oz) dairy milk, or nut milk of choice

FOR THE GLAZE

25 g (1 oz) butter, melted
60 g (2¼ oz) icing (confectioners') sugar, sifted
2 teaspoons dairy milk, or nut milk of choice
¼ teaspoon ground cinnamon
pinch of ground ginger
pinch of ground turmeric
pinch of ground cardamom
¼ teaspoon vanilla extract

Preheat the oven to 180°C (350°F), Gas Mark 4 and line a muffin tray with 8 paper cases (cups).

Cream the butter and sugar in a large bowl with a wooden spoon until pale and fluffy. Gradually add the egg and vanilla extract and mix together until fully incorporated.

In a separate bowl, combine all the dry ingredients including the spices. Add half the dry ingredients to the egg and sugar mixture and stir until fully combined. Add half the milk and mix in before adding the remaining dry ingredients. Finally, incorporate the rest of the milk and beat until you have a smooth mixture.

Spoon this mixture into each muffin case almost to the top. Bake for 20–25 minutes, or until the tops of the muffins are well risen and spring back when touched (or check with a skewer). Transfer to a wire rack to cool.

Meanwhile, combine all the glaze ingredients in a bowl until smooth. Once the muffins have cooled for 5–10 minutes, dip their tops into the glaze and set aside until it hardens. They can then be double-dipped if desired for extra flavour. Alternatively, you can drizzle the glaze over the tops of the muffins with a spoon.

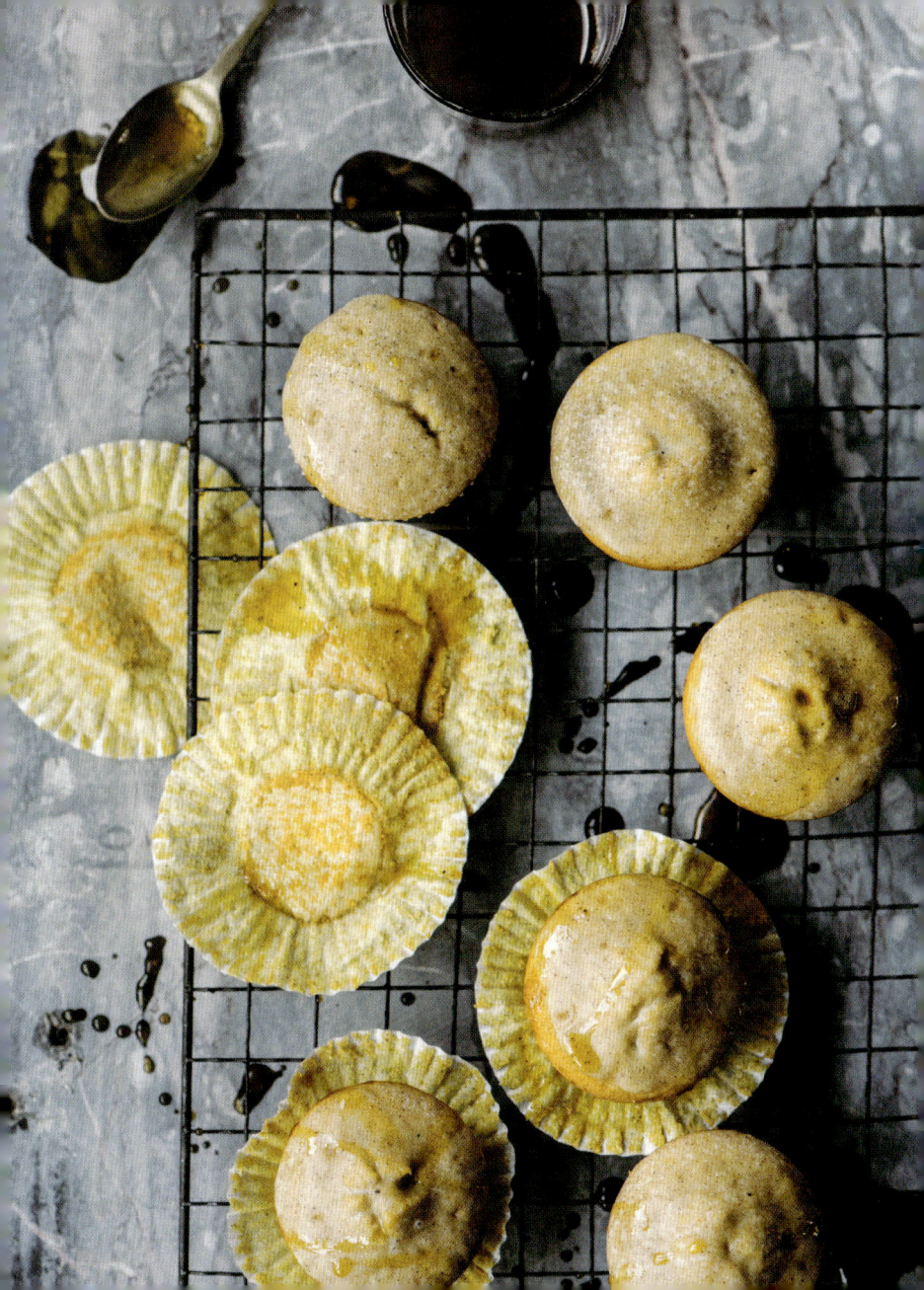

SERVES 2

TURMERIC-GLAZED BANANA
with ice cream

Here we have the simplest of desserts. The turmeric complements the sweetness of the banana and maple syrup to give just the right balance.

- 2 tablespoons unsalted butter
- 1 teaspoon grated fresh turmeric
- 1 large or 2 small bananas, peeled and sliced in half lengthways
- 2 tablespoons maple syrup
- 2 scoops of vanilla ice cream or coconut yogurt

Place a large frying pan (skillet) over a medium heat and add the butter. When bubbling hot, add the turmeric followed by the bananas, cut-side down. Allow to colour in the butter and turmeric for a couple of minutes, then add the maple syrup to thicken the sauce.

Serve hot with a scoop of vanilla ice cream or coconut yogurt on the side.

SERVES 6

COCONUT RICE PUDDING
with turmeric, lemon grass & ginger syrup

A variation on the traditional rice pudding, this recipe simply adds coconut, turmeric, lemon grass and ginger to make it spiced and sweet at the same time.

---

2 x 400 ml (14 fl oz) cans coconut milk
200 ml (7 fl oz) water
130 g (4 oz) arborio or basmati rice, washed and drained
110 g (3¾ oz) palm sugar or soft light brown sugar
1 lemon grass stalk, ends trimmed and outer layers discarded

FOR THE SYRUP
375 ml (13 fl oz) water
1 teaspoon ground turmeric
2 lemon grass stalks, prepared as above
2.5 cm (1 in) piece of stem ginger, thickly sliced into 4
pared rind of 1 lime, plus juice
pinch of ground black pepper
80 g (3 oz) palm sugar or soft light brown sugar

TO GARNISH
apple blossom flowers
few sprigs of lemon verbena

Start by making the syrup. Put the water, turmeric, lemon grass, ginger, lime rind and pepper in a small saucepan and bring to the boil. Reduce to a simmer and let the syrup bubble away for 5–10 minutes, or until reduced by half.

Once reduced, strain the syrup into a bowl, discarding the contents of the sieve. Return the syrup to the pan, add the sugar and bring to the boil. Reduce for about 5 minutes, until a syrupy consistency is achieved. Cool the syrup, then add 1–2 teaspoons of lime juice to taste. Set the syrup aside.

Put the coconut milk and water in a medium pan and bring to the boil, then add the rice, sugar and lemon grass, stirring well. As soon as the liquid returns to the boil, reduce the heat to medium and cook the rice slowly for about 20 minutes, stirring occasionally so as not to burn the bottom of the pan. Once the rice is cooked but still al dente, take the pan off the heat and discard the lemon grass stalk.

Serve the rice pudding warm or cold, topped with a spoonful of the spiced syrup and garnished with apple blossom flowers and lemon verbena sprigs, if liked.

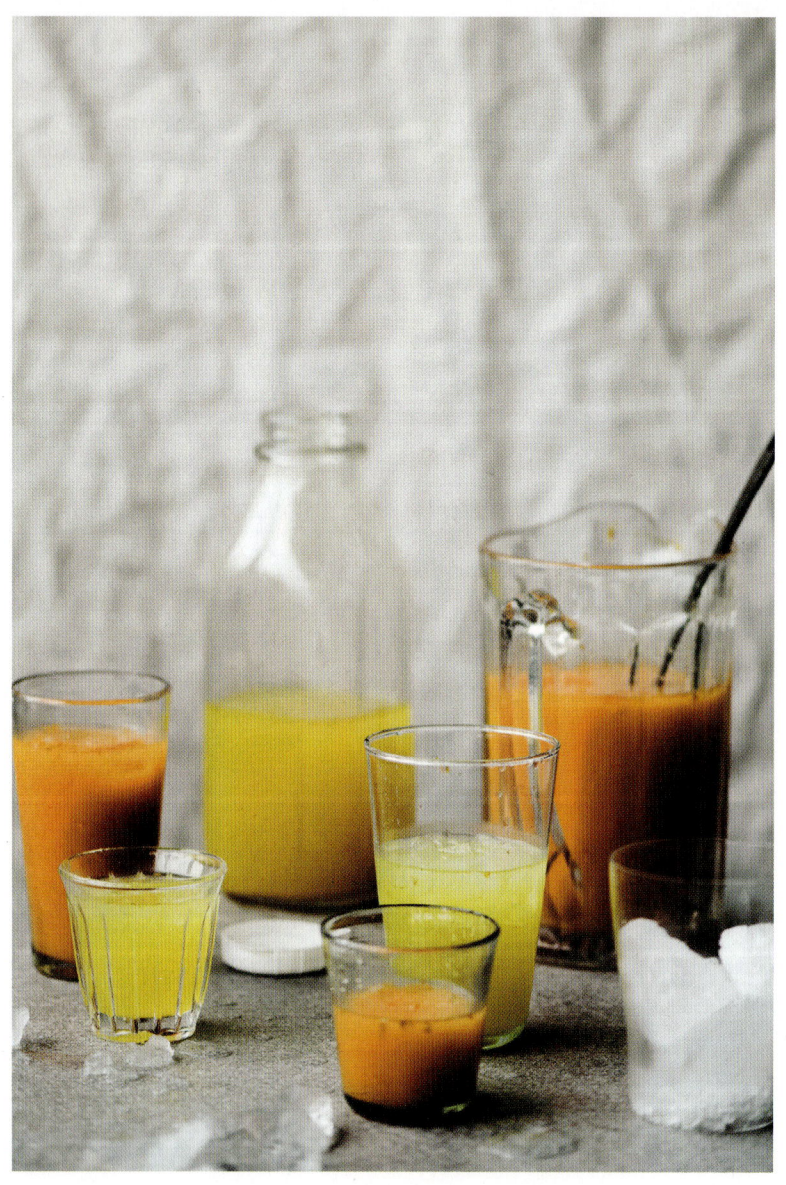

MAKES 750 ML (1¼ PINTS)

APPLE TURMERIC TONIC

For an extra shot of goodness, add a few drops of holy basil tincture, an adaptogen that helps your body to cope better with stress.

---

750 ml (1¼ pints) pressed apple juice
3 teaspoons grated fresh turmeric
3 teaspoons grated fresh root ginger
juice of 2 lemons

Put all the ingredients into a large jug or bowl and allow the flavours to infuse for a few hours, or overnight if possible.

Strain into a large glass bottle. Chill in the refrigerator, where it will keep for up to 3 days. Give the bottle a good shake before serving.

MAKES 500 ML (17 FL OZ)

TURMERIC TODDY

Thyme is good for relieving a sore throat, and combines well with the ginger, turmeric, honey and lime in this drink, which boosts your immune system.

---

10 g (¼ oz) fresh thyme sprigs
1 cm (½ in) piece of fresh root ginger, peeled and grated
1 teaspoon grated fresh turmeric or ground turmeric
¼ teaspoon black peppercorns
500 ml (17 fl oz) water
2 tablespoons raw honey
juice of 1 lime

Use a rolling pin to lightly bash the thyme, which will help to release its oil.

Add the thyme, ginger, turmeric, peppercorns and measured water to a saucepan and bring to just below the boil. Reduce the heat and simmer for 10 minutes.

Remove from the heat and add the honey and lime juice, stirring until the honey is dissolved. Strain and serve.

MAKES 1 LARGE POT

TURMERIC TEA

A wonderfully refreshing tea, this is perfect for starting the day with, or as a pick-me-up in the afternoon. The addition of cinnamon makes it lovely and warming, although you could replace this with a teaspoon of green tea leaves. For even more of a chai taste, replace the lemon grass with a few cloves and bashed cardamom pods.

---

1 litre (1¾ pints) water
½ cinnamon stick
1 lemon grass stalk, bashed
few slices of fresh root ginger
few slices of fresh turmeric
   or 1 heaped teaspoon ground
   turmeric
¼ teaspoon black peppercorns

Pour the measured water into a large saucepan and bring to the boil.

Gradually mix in the herbs and spices, then simmer gently for 10 minutes.

Strain into a teapot and serve.

SERVES 1

GOLDEN MYLK

A traditional drink enjoyed in Indonesia, you can try it with or without the cinnamon, maple syrup or honey, depending on your taste.

---

300 ml (½ pint) almond or
   coconut milk
½ teaspoon ground turmeric
½ teaspoon ground cinnamon
pinch of ground black pepper
1 teaspoon coconut oil
1 teaspoon maple syrup or honey

Put the almond or coconut milk into a pan and warm gently over a low heat.

Meanwhile, put the remaining ingredients in a small bowl, add a little boiled water and stir to make a paste. Whisk this into the warming milk, then continue to heat gently for 5 minutes. It's then ready to serve.

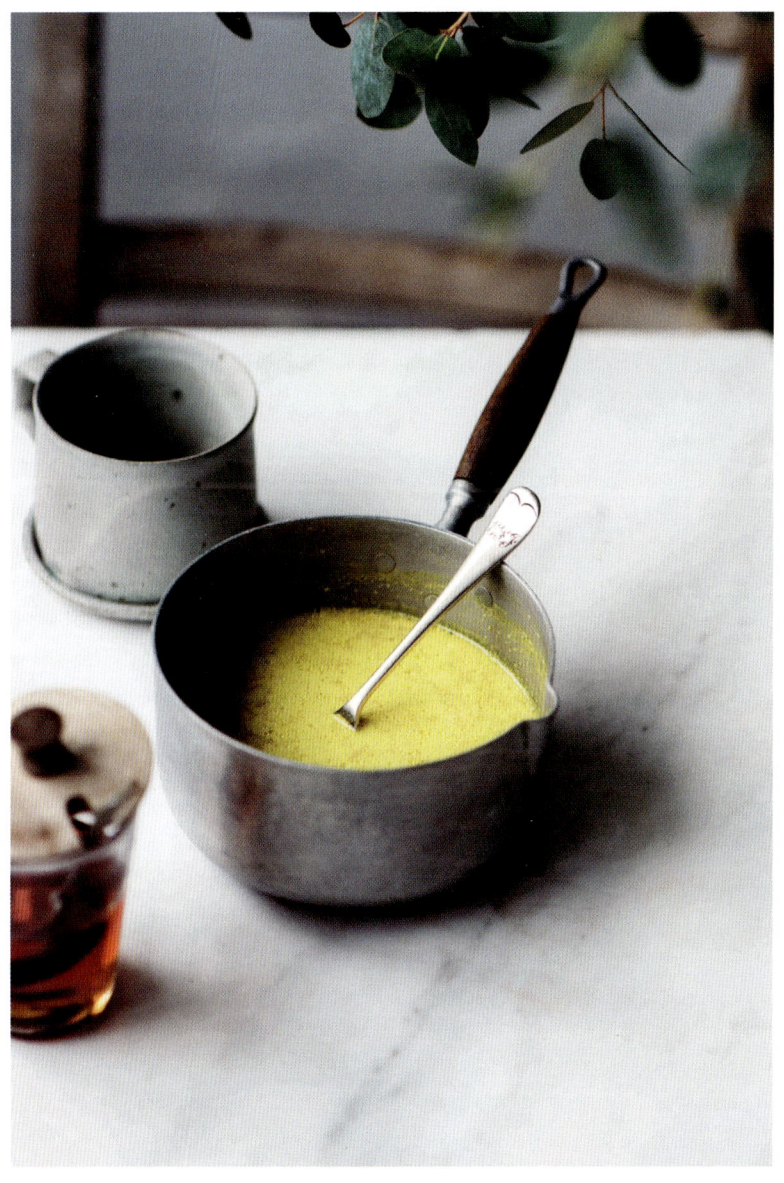

INDEX

almond milk
  golden mylk 76
apple
  apple turmeric tonic 75
  Bircher muesli with turmeric honey 11
  turmeric bliss balls 28
aubergines
  aubergine with tofu & turmeric dengaku 39
avocado
  scrambled eggs with avocado on toast 14

bacon & egg-drop miso 23
bananas
  turmeric banana bread 40
  turmeric-glazed banana with ice cream 72
beans
  Buddha bowl 50
  kitchari 21
beef stew 62
bhindi masala curry 52
Bircher muesli with turmeric honey 11
biscuits
  turmeric maple ice cream 69
bread
  scrambled eggs with avocado on toast 14
broccoli
  roast chicken with tandoori rub 64
Buddha bowl 50
bulgur
  sweet potato bulgur 46
butter
  corn on the cob with turmeric butter 35

carrots
  beef stew 62
  ginger & turmeric carrot soup 19
cashew nuts
  coconut & cashew granola 12
cauliflower
  roast cauliflower salad 49

cavolo nero
  frittata 13
  miso turmeric glazed salmon 56
chai muffins, turmeric 70
cheese
  frittata 13
  turmeric gnocchi 53
  yellow rice with coconut halloumi 45
chicken
  coconut chicken soup with turmeric & kale 26
  roast chicken with tandoori rub 64
chickpeas
  five veg tagine 47
  turmeric hummus 33
chillies
  mussels with turmeric & lemon grass 61
  rasam with sashimi & wilting greens 25
cinnamon
  golden mylk 76
  turmeric tea 76
coconut
  coconut & cashew granola 12
  coconut chicken soup with turmeric & kale 26
  squash & coconut dhal 22
  turmeric bliss balls 28
  yellow rice with coconut halloumi 45
coconut milk
  coconut rice pudding 73
  golden mylk 76
  aubergine with tofu & turmeric dengaku 39
cod
  Keralan fish curry 59
  turmeric & tamarind cod 60
corn on the cob with turmeric butter 35
cream
  turmeric maple ice cream 69
cucumber
  turmeric & tamarind cod 60

eggs
- bacon & egg-drop miso — 23
- scrambled eggs with avocado on toast — 14
- frittata — 13

fish
- Keralan fish curry — 59
- miso turmeric glazed salmon — 56
- smoked mackerel turmeric congee — 16
- turmeric & tamarind cod — 60

five veg tagine — 47
frittata — 13

ginger
- apple turmeric tonic — 75
- coconut rice pudding — 73
- ginger & turmeric carrot soup — 19
- roast cauliflower salad — 49
- turmeric tea — 76
- turmeric toddy — 75

granola — 12

hazelnuts
- Bircher muesli with turmeric honey — 11

honey
- Bircher muesli with turmeric honey — 11
- coconut & cashew granola — 12
- turmeric & tamarind cod — 60
- turmeric bliss balls — 28
- turmeric toddy — 75

hummus, turmeric — 33

ice cream
- turmeric maple ice cream — 69
- turmeric-glazed banana with ice cream — 72

kale
- coconut chicken soup with turmeric & kale — 26
- rasam with sashimi & wilting greens — 25
- aubergine with tofu & turmeric dengaku — 39
- sweet potato bulgur — 46

kitchari — 21

lemon grass
- coconut rice pudding — 73
- mussels with turmeric & lemon grass — 61
- turmeric tea — 76

lemons
- apple turmeric tonic — 75

limes
- Bircher muesli with turmeric honey — 11
- roast cauliflower salad — 49
- turmeric toddy — 75

mackerel
- smoked mackerel turmeric congee — 16

maple syrup
- golden mylk — 76
- turmeric maple ice cream — 69
- turmeric-glazed banana with ice cream — 72

miso
- bacon & egg-drop miso — 23
- miso turmeric glazed salmon — 56

muesli
- Bircher muesli with turmeric honey — 11

muffins
- turmeric chai muffins — 70

mushrooms
- Buddha bowl — 50

mussels with turmeric & lemon grass — 61
mustard, turmeric — 43

oats
- Bircher muesli with turmeric honey — 11
- coconut & cashew granola — 12
- turmeric & black pepper oatcakes — 31

oil, turmeric-infused — 43

okra
- bhindi masala curry — 52

onions
- beef stew — 62
- kitchari — 21

pak choi
- miso turmeric glazed salmon — 56

pasta
  turmeric prawn linguine 55
peas, split
  squash & coconut dhal 22
pepper, black
  turmeric & black pepper oatcakes 31
pickles, turmeric 42
popcorn 67
potatoes
  potato salad with turmeric tahini dressing 36
  turmeric gnocchi 53
prawns
  turmeric prawn linguine 55

quinoa
  roast cauliflower salad 49

rasam with sashimi & wilting greens 25
rice
  Buddha bowl 50
  coconut rice pudding 73
  Keralan fish curry 59
  rice with coconut halloumi 45
  smoked mackerel turmeric congee 16

salmon
  miso turmeric glazed salmon 56
  rasam with sashimi & wilting greens 25
seafood
  mussels with turmeric & lemon grass 61
  turmeric prawn
    linguine 55
seaweed
  kitchari 21
  turmeric gnocchi 53
seeds
  Bircher muesli with turmeric honey 11
  coconut & cashew granola 12
  kitchari 21
  spiced & roasted seeds 30

spices
  scrambled eggs with avocado on toast 14
  popcorn 67
  roast chicken with tandoori rub 64
  spiced & roasted seeds 30
  turmeric chai muffins 70
spinach
  Keralan fish curry 59
  rasam with sashimi & wilting greens 25
squash & coconut dhal 22
sweet potato bulgur 46

tahini
  potato salad with turmeric tahini dressing 36
tamarind
  turmeric & tamarind cod 60
tea
  turmeric tea 76
thyme
  turmeric toddy 75
tofu
  Buddha bowl 50
  aubergine with tofu & turmeric dengaku 39
tomatoes
  bhindi masala curry 52
  turmeric prawn linguine 55
turnips
  beef stew 62

vegetables
  Buddha bowl 50
  five veg tagine 47
  turmeric pickles 42

yogurt
  Bircher muesli with turmeric honey 11
  turmeric prawn linguine 55